Nutrition Policy in Canada, 1870-1939

Aleck Samuel Ostry

Nutrition Policy in Canada, 1870-1939

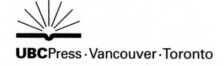

UBCPress · Vancouver · Toronto

15 14 13 12 11 10 09 08 07 06   5 4 3 2 1

Printed in Canada on ancient-forest-free paper (100% post-consumer recycled)
that is processed chlorine- and acid-free, with vegetable-based inks.

Library and Archives Canada Cataloguing in Publication

Ostry, Aleck Samuel, 1952-
   Nutrition policy in Canada, 1870-1939 / Aleck Samuel Ostry.

Includes bibliographical references and index.
ISBN: 978-0-7748-1327-3 (bound); 978-0-7748-1328-0 (pbk)

   1. Nutrition policy – Canada – History. 2. Food industry and trade – Canada –
Safety measures – History. 3. Food industry and trade – Standards – Canada –
History. I. Title.

TX360.C3O96 2006   363.80971   C2006-905180-1

Canadä

UBC Press gratefully acknowledges the financial support for our publishing
program of the Government of Canada through the Book Publishing Industry
Development Program (BPIDP), and of the Canada Council for the Arts, and the
British Columbia Arts Council.

This book has been published with the help of a grant from the Canadian
Federation for the Humanities and Social Sciences, through the Aid to Scholarly
Publications Programme, using funds provided by the Social Sciences and
Humanities Research Council of Canada, and with the help of the K.D.
Srivastava Fund.

UBC Press
The University of British Columbia
2029 West Mall
Vancouver, BC V6T 1Z2
604-822-5959 / Fax: 604-822-6083
www.ubcpress.ca

This book is dedicated to my parents.

Contents

Figures and Tables

Acknowledgments

I would like to acknowledge the support of the Canadian Institutes for Health Research (CIHR) and the Michael Smith Foundation for Health Research in British Columbia (MSFHR). In 2000 I obtained a five-year CIHR New Investigator award and in 2002 a five-year MSFHR scholar award. Both of these awards paid my salary. Without their support this work would not have been possible.

Finally, several people helped me research this book. I'd like to thank Tara Shannon, Merrilee Hughes, and, particularly, Tasnim Nathoo for their assistance. Also, Graham Riches, after reading the manuscript, gave me very useful advice on how to improve it further. As well, after I submitted the initial manuscript to UBC Press, two anonymous reviewers gave me useful feedback, which I used to substantially improve this work. While this help is acknowledged and appreciated, in the final analysis this book is my responsibility. Any errors in omission or commission are mine alone.

Nutrition Policy in Canada, 1870-1939

Introduction

As nations industrialized and began to grapple with feeding urbanized populations, the increasing separation of people from the land and their concentration in big cities led to the establishment of vast systems of food production, distribution, storage, and sale – systems that were largely governed by private markets. In most nations government stepped in during the late nineteenth century to regulate these markets, at first solely to ensure economic order but later also to protect human health.

Today most states have complex legal and regulatory systems that monitor food production at all levels. Scientists establish standards that regulate the content of food and design programs of health promotion and education in order to disseminate nutritional information. As well, a complex industry grows, processes, distributes, sells, and trades food, sometimes openly but often in a highly protected manner.

Today public interest in food and nutrition (ranging from broad worries about the sustainability and safety of systems of agricultural production to the desire for information on the links between vitamin intake and specific diseases) is very high. The public's interest in the relationship between food, diet, and health has not always been this intense. It has waxed and waned. For example, during the economic hardships of the Depression worries about the links between malnutrition and ill health, particularly among the children of the unemployed, was high. With a full-employment economy following the Second World War, and for two decades thereafter, until links between high fat diets and coronary heart disease became widely known, the public's interest in food and health waned in Canada.

Now, however, consumers are hungry for health news, particularly about fitness and nutrition. Newspapers, television, and the Internet have steadily increased their coverage of health issues (Pellechia 1997). In a recent study more than 70 percent of the science coverage in three major American newspapers was health-related (American Readership Institute Survey 2001). While most of this health news dealt with the etiology and treatments of diseases, including food-borne illness, the second most common area of health coverage was lifestyle, which, in turn, was dominated by issues of weight loss.

While in most developed nations the print and broadcast media have, historically, been the major sources of health and nutrition information for the public (Begley and Cardwell 1996; Goldberg 1997, 2000), two major changes are under way in the Canadian media. Most television stations now have specialized reporters and increasingly large segments of news casts devoted to "health news." The use of the Internet has increased, as has the proliferation of health- and nutrition-focused Web sites (Goldberg 2000). Compared to other developed nations Canada has among the highest Internet access and use rates in the world, and in 2000 and 2001 health sites accounted for 13 percent of the total online media sites used by all Canadians (Media Metrix 2000, 2001). In Canada the subject of nutritional health is the fastest-growing area of interest on the Internet (Kouris-Blazos et al. 2001).

While people thirst for information about nutrition and health, it is not clear that reading newspapers, watching television, and surfing the Internet will meet their needs. For example, according to the few studies that have been conducted, nutrition information available on the Internet is of low reliability and accuracy both in the United States (Miles et al. 2000) and in Canada (Davison and Guan 1996). Often, media articles and news on nutrition and health describe single studies, with limited context provided in "sound-bite" style, so that people have a difficult time developing a clear understanding of the relationship between nutrition and health.

Thus, the public is left with disconnected tidbits of information (often biased by the interests of industry and various disease- or nutrition-based foundations and institutes) that do not add up to a coherent whole and do not allow for the development of a nuanced, "big-picture" view of the relationship between nutrition and health, on the one hand, and the structure and process of nutrition policy making and health on the other. Without information on the latter, people don't know how to become involved in, or otherwise influence, the policy process in ways that might improve either food security or their own nutritional status.

The combination of a growth in public interest in the links between nutrition and health within a context of increased concern about the health effects of diet (particularly from overeating); the media proliferation of unreliable information on nutrition and health (and the increasing power of consumers to find this information on the Internet); and the growing commercial stake in marketing food based on health claims (and an increasingly lenient regulatory environment) is a recipe for public confusion. In Canada this problem is exacerbated by a lack of basic historical research on nutrition policy, the links between nutrition and health, and how these have changed over time. This research is essential to current policy-making efforts.

One could divide the history of nutrition policy in Canada into five main eras. The first era, lasting roughly from the mid-1870s to the end of the First World War, was dominated by the establishment of a system of food safety, inspection, and surveillance. This system was developed within the framework of federal criminal law, and its purpose was to counter widespread food adulteration in order to protect consumers from economic fraud and to preserve the integrity of the trade in food.

The second era of nutrition policy occurred during the interwar years, and it saw a more activist federal government begin to use its spending power in areas of social and health (including nutrition) policy, which were formally under provincial jurisdiction (Ostry 2006). The establishment of the federal Department of Health in 1919 marked the beginning of this period, and the formation of the Canadian Council on Nutrition in 1938 marked its end.

For several reasons nutritional policy issues in the 1920s were different from those in the past. A spate of new vitamin research throughout the 1920s linked a deficiency in certain vitamins with diseases such as rickets. The discovery of vitamins caught the public imagination, drawing increased attention to the relationship between nutrition and health. These developments occurred as the new retail chain stores expanded through mass advertising.

As well, in the 1920s, when the supply of cow's milk was uneven and the milk itself of uncertain quality in most regions of Canada, nutrition policy makers directed their attention towards breastfeeding. Accordingly, the first national nutrition policies specifically related to improving the health of Canadians (and largely ignored by Canadian mothers until the late 1960s) were developed by the federal Department of Health in order to promote breastfeeding.

As the Depression worsened in the early 1930s widespread unemployment put the issue of hunger squarely on the public policy agenda. The debate was highly politicized as malnutrition and dietary standards became central to an increasingly intense political struggle regarding appropriate relief payments for the unemployed. By the end of the decade the focus of nutrition policy making had shifted to the development of a national dietary standard. This was part of an international effort in which the League of Nations aggressively promoted the new nutrition science and its application to problems of global unemployment and stagnating agricultural trade.

The 1930s were also important because this was when the medical profession consolidated its role as a major stakeholder in nutrition education, particularly in relation to infant feeding. The profession, particularly pediatrics, had helped to develop and market the first commercial artificial baby foods. Its involvement in dispensing infant feeding advice to new mothers accelerated as, beginning in the early 1930s, birthing increasingly shifted from home to hospital.

The third era of nutrition policy making spanned the lifetime of the Canadian Council on Nutrition (CCN), from 1938 to 1972. This institution, along with the Nutrition Services Division of the federal Department of Health and the Department of Agriculture, shaped wartime dietary standards and ensured that key workers (e.g., munitions workers and other producers of essential war equipment and goods) were well fed.

From the 1950s through the 1970s the CCN developed national policies on food fortification in conjunction with the Department of Health as various elements and vitamins were added to the Canadian food supply. Ironically, during this time of growing agricultural production, increased access to and consumption of food, and even early warnings of an emerging obesity problem, nutrition policy making (especially fortification policies) continued to be driven largely by Depression-era concerns over malnutrition, particularly in relation to vitamin and mineral deficiencies.

As the life of the CCN came to an end, one of its last acts was the coordination of the world's first representative national dietary survey. In 1972 the results of this huge survey were published. It demonstrated some nutrient deficiencies, particularly among young women, that were blamed partly on restrained eating and dieting. Most important, the survey noted that, in Canada, being overweight was an "epidemic problem," that this was an extremely difficult nutritional problem to correct, and that it had been a problem in Canada likely since the 1950s (Beaton 1981).

The fourth era in nutrition policy making lasted from the demise of the CCN in 1973 to the publication of modern dietary guidelines in 1992. The beginning of this era witnessed the end of the post-Second World War economic expansion and, in the mid- and late 1970s, serious food price inflation. After almost a quarter century of relative public unconcern about nutrition and its links with health, the 1970s witnessed new citizen activism and government policy making as worries grew that the poor unemployed might lack food.

This was also when Ancel Keys's (1970) groundbreaking research linking dietary fat intake and coronary heart disease began to be taken seriously by the public and by some nutrition and health policy makers. As well, in the 1970s and 1980s nutrition policy making in the federal Department of Health was dominated by the health promotion paradigm, first outlined in the Lalonde Report (Lalonde 1974). Framed within this model, nutrition policy making shifted almost completely to a reliance on the twin pillars of nutrition education (which was also increasingly well coordinated with provincial ministries of health) and food fortification.

The fifth (and current) era of nutrition policy making, under way since the early 1990s, has been marked by the consolidation and internationalization of the agrifood sector. Since the signing of the North American Free Trade Agreement and the birth of the World Trade Organization, the new North American and global trade environment has accelerated the integration of national agribusiness sectors on a hemispheric and global level, increasing pressure to internationalize food standards and dietary guidelines and to dismantle supply management and other so-called hidden tariffs in Canada. And this has occurred as biotechnology has evolved to allow genetic manipulation of the food supply.

While I have framed the history of nutrition policy in Canada from the late nineteenth century to the present within five eras, the focus of this book is on the first two, from the 1870s to 1939. These two periods saw a shift in agricultural production from grains to meats, the birth of modern nutrition science, the increasing involvement of the medical profession in advising people about nutrition and health, and the establishment of a national nutrition policy-making institution.

These two eras of nutrition policy making in Canada have remained underinvestigated. As well, the federal policy-making institutions that drove nutrition policy in the 1950s and 1960s – primarily the Nutrition Services Division of the Department of Health and the Canadian Council on Nutrition – were profoundly shaped by developments in politics, science, health, and agriculture, all of which occurred before these institutions were established on the eve of the Second World War. The political and scientific debates and priorities concerning food and health during this time comprised the foundation around which most of the early nutrition policies and nutrition policy-making institutions were formed. Understanding foundational developments during this period is important because they continued to influence nutrition policy making for decades after the Second World War, in particular as the Depression-era thinking about undernutrition continued to dominate nutrition policy making even as overnutrition and obesity were becoming national problems.[1]

In most areas of health and social policy the federal government used its spending power to shape provincial and national policy (Ostry 2006). However, in the case of nutrition policy prior to the Second World War the federal government took a more direct lead. The earliest federal foray into nutrition policy was through the Adulteration Act, which was framed within federal criminal law. This act and the food safety system upon which it is based was not (at least at first) about health and, therefore, was not a provincial constitutional responsibility.

As well, after 1919 and the passage of the federal Department of Health Act, the federal government was mandated to coordinate "efforts for preserving and improving public health, conservation of child life and promotion of child welfare" (Canada 1919). Thus, public health efforts to improve the nutritional health of infants and children became a direct federal responsibility, which is partly why the first national nutritional guidelines were developed in relation to breastfeeding.

The federal government was also aggressively and indirectly involved in nutrition education through the activities of the Department of Agriculture, which became heavily involved in promoting milk consumption among children from the 1920s onwards. And, in the 1930s, establishment of a national dietary standard became an important element of a government strategy to reform national labour policy and the delivery of unemployment insurance (Grauer 1939; Struthers 1983).

---

[1] There is evidence that, as early as 1945, nutritionists were beginning to worry about overweight and obesity in the Canadian population (Beaton 1981; Pett 1972). For example, in summarizing the overall results of the limited number of (albeit unrepresentative) dietary surveys conducted between the early 1930s and 1950 (with approximately 10,000 individuals), Pett (1972) observed that, in some surveys, overweight was found in up to 33 percent of respondents. And Beaton (1981), commenting on the results of the 1972 nutrition survey, claimed the obesity was a problem of epidemic proportion. As well, as early as 1945 there is evidence of concern that inflated dietary standards encouraged overeating. At present, nutritionists and public health experts appear to be unaware that overweight and obesity (albeit not as severe at present and not as severe among children) has been a problem since the 1950s.

This book focuses on three basic themes in nutrition policy between the 1870s and the beginning of the Second World War: (1) food adulteration and the evolution of a system of food safety, inspection, and surveillance; (2) policies on breastfeeding; and (3) the scientific and policy developments leading to a national dietary standard. The context of these three themes is key to achieving a nuanced historical understanding of nutrition policy. Accordingly, I examine this context in light of four subthemes.

The first subtheme involves early nutrition policies that were focused mainly on milk. In the late nineteenth century milk was the most widely adulterated food in Canada. Indeed, it was known as a dangerous food that killed babies. Beginning in the 1920s, and bolstered by the discovery of vitamins, milk underwent a fundamental makeover and was increasingly touted as the quintessential "protective food" for children. In the 1930s the price of milk and milk marketing were major economic and health issues. Thus, the changing scientific and public image and the marketing of milk was central to the nutritional health of infants in Canada during this time.

The second subtheme involves the changing nutritional and health status of the Canadian population from the 1870s to the beginning of the Second World War. Especially after 1919 nutritional policy was driven by concerns about the links between poverty, malnutrition, and ill health (particularly among infants).

The third subtheme involves the medical profession's role in dispensing nutritional advice, which emerged slowly and steadily throughout the nineteenth century. By the beginning of the Second World War physicians were trusted experts who were increasingly consulted by governments with regard to developing nutrition policy. As well, the interaction between the medical profession, the government, and ordinary (particularly female) citizens is key to gaining a better understanding of how breastfeeding policy and dietary standards were shaped.

Finally, while the federal Department of Agriculture had always been a powerful player in Canadian history (MacRae 1999), its indirect and usually underacknowledged role in shaping nutrition education (particularly through its marketing branch) became more important as the industry faced crippling economic pressure in the 1930s. Beginning in the 1920s the agricultural industry and the Department of Agriculture helped to shape nutritional health policy, both directly and indirectly, through their alliances with the federal Department of Health and through their explicit use of health-based claims to promote sales of Canadian agricultural products. Today, this interaction between health and agricultural interests remains key to understanding nutrition policy development.

This book has nine chapters. The first three cover the period from the 1870s to 1920; the next two cover the 1920s; and the remaining four focus on the 1930s. Chapter 1 identifies the origins of Canada's food safety legislation and the subsequent evolution of the national food surveillance system. I describe food safety laws during colonial times as well as the origins of Canadian legislation in British criminal law. Chapter 2 evaluates the evidence relating to the nutritional status of the population prior to the First World War. It also outlines the problem of persistently high infant mortality rates as this issue shaped the breast-feeding guidelines that were developed after the war. Chapter 3 moves from the consideration of the food safety system outlined in Chapter 1 to a discussion of the safety of artificial infant foods as these emerged in the late nineteenth century, championed by the new medical specialty of pediatrics.

Chapter 4 describes the changing image of cow's milk as, with new vitamin discoveries, it was transformed from unhealthy liquid into the perfect food for children. This transformation is key to the infant feeding guidelines developed in the 1920s, which are outlined in detail in Chapter 5.

Chapters 6 to 8 focus on the 1930s. Chapter 6 shifts back to food safety, picking up where Chapter 1 left off in 1920 and continuing to 1939. The combination of new techniques of food production and marketing in the 1920s, the growing popularity of vitamins, and the potential for false health claims fraud (compounded by the worsening economic crisis of the 1930s) created new food surveillance and monitoring problems for the federal Department of Health. The Depression also altered the agricultural sector's approach to marketing food as the industry struggled with closed export markets and persistently low prices. The final section in this chapter revisits the role of the medical profession in dispensing nutrition advice during the 1930s.

Chapter 7 utilizes the available evidence to assess the nutritional and dietary status of Canadians during the 1930s. This issue framed the debates linking nutrition, unemployment, and the creation of the 1938 dietary standard. Chapter 8 outlines the changes in mortality due to nutritional deficiency diseases as a crude indicator of the extent of hunger and its impact on health during this decade of economic hardship. Chapter 9 describes the origins of the 1938 dietary standard, the establishment of the Canadian Council on Nutrition, and the role the League of Nations played in its formation. The final chapter summarizes findings and presents conclusions.

I used seven types of sources in conducting the research for this book. First, I consulted general historical works. Second, I reviewed books and articles on agricultural policy and agricultural economics in late nineteenth- and early twentieth-century Canada. Third, I studied the few books exploring nutrition policy in Canadian history. Investigations in this area are limited (e.g., there are only two main works [Curran 1954; Davidson 1949] on the development of the food safety system in Canada from the 1870s to the 1930s). In order to supplement these sources, I obtained federal Department of Health and Department of Agriculture reports to determine "official" views on nutrition issues. Fifth, from Statistics Canada I obtained data on national food disappearance, food consumption, and food prices as well as data on infant mortality and nutritional deficiency diseases mortality. Sixth, through the Ottawa Historical Archives, I obtained minutes of meetings of the Canadian Council on Nutrition. Although the council was formed in 1938, the minutes cover events that occurred from the early-1930s onward. Finally, I systematically scanned late nineteenth- and early twentieth-century nutrition and medical journals such as the *Canadian Public Health Journal* in order to obtain information on the development of pediatrics, advice about infant feeding, and the results of early dietary surveys.

The provinces have played an obvious and important role in developing nutrition policy. A more detailed historical review of the provincial role is beyond the scope of this book but should undoubtedly be undertaken as the differences in the development of nutrition policy across regions may prove a fruitful arena for historical and current studies of food security and nutrition policy.

1
Establishing a Food Surveillance System in Canada

Prior to 1919 and the establishment of the federal Department of Health, nutrition policy was shaped mainly by the Adulteration Act, 1874. As Canada's first consumer protection law, it was designed to shield food purchasers from fraud due to the deliberate adulteration of food, which usually occurred when food wholesalers and retailers added contaminants and fillers in order to increase profits. This was a common (almost accepted) business practice in the late nineteenth century.

Under the authority of the Adulteration Act, inspection facilities, laboratories, and an inspectorate were organized and began to operate nationwide by 1919. The Adulteration Act was framed within criminal law, and its purpose was to police food manufacturers, distributors, and retailers in order to prevent economic fraud. Thus, by the late nineteenth century the federal government was playing a role in nutritional health.

This chapter describes the early development of a system of food safety and shows why and how the federal government became involved in nutrition policy making. It explains the origins and subsequent evolution of the Adulteration Act and is divided into four sections. The first section describes food laws enacted by the French and British colonial regimes; the second section reviews the origins of the British food adulteration legislation, upon which the original Canadian legislation was based; the third section describes the conditions in Canada that led to the passage of this legislation; and the last section describes how, by the end of the First World War, the federal government had established a national food surveillance regimen.

Food Laws during the Colonial Period
During the French regime food laws were enacted to cope with periodic scarcity as, at various times during the sixteenth and seventeenth

centuries, the fledgling colony was threatened with crop failure and, during the first half of the eighteenth century, with British blockades. As well, in the quarter century prior to the British conquest, the French colonial administration was particularly corrupt. Royal officials often manipulated prices, particularly of imported food, in order to extract personal gain, thus creating hardships for the colonists (McLynn 2005).

In New France there were several instances when rationing and price controls were implemented because of poor harvests and military blockades. For example, following a crop failure in 1713 a regulation was passed prohibiting grain exports and forcing farmers to sell most of their grain (after keeping enough for their families) to bakers, who could use it only for baking bread (Davidson 1949).

As the colony became more agriculturally self-sufficient emergency laws designed to avoid food scarcity were enacted less frequently; instead, regulations were passed to control grading, storage conditions, and weights and volumes of staple food items such as fish, pork, sugar, flour, and butter. Similar laws were enacted by the British following the conquest of New France, and under British rule a small inspectorate was soon established to control food adulteration (Davidson 1949).

The Adulteration Act, 1874, was modelled directly on England's Adulteration of Food and Drugs Act, 1872. It is therefore to England that we must briefly turn in order to better understand the origins of Canada's modern food legislation.

Influence of British Legislation

The earliest British food legislation was the 1266 Assize of Bread and Ale statute, which imposed standard weights for a loaf of bread and volume standards for ale (Fallows 1988). Between the thirteenth and eighteenth centuries food laws, mainly controlling weights and measures, were enacted on an ad hoc basis and mainly in towns where the guilds were powerful enough to police them. In the early eighteenth century local standards for the weight and price of bread were legislated and enforced by magistrates. Additional legislation was passed in 1757 to prevent adulteration and to specify permitted ingredients for bread. The purpose of these early bread laws was to create a level marketplace for bakers rather than to ensure consumer protection (Fallows 1988).

In the early nineteenth century the industrial revolution uprooted millions of farmers and agricultural labourers, turning them into landless city dwellers. During this time new food manufacturing industries and distribution facilities were created to serve the rapidly growing urban population. There is some evidence that adulteration of food, by both manufacturers and retailers, was widespread and largely tolerated by the authorities (Jukes 1987).

However, during the nineteenth century several new developments began to alter the laissez-faire public and official attitudes towards food adulteration. By the 1820s advances in chemistry made it possible to detect common adulterants in food and led to the publication of the first "Treatise on the Adulteration of Food and Culinary Poisons," in which evidence of food adulteration was demonstrated using the latest analytic techniques (Hassall 1855). By the 1860s these new skills had greatly enhanced the prestige of chemists and provided the state with the technical capacity to detect many common food adulterants.

As well, by mid-century public health professionals and citizens had forged a coalition that pressured the British Parliament to enact the world's first public health laws. This legislation laid the foundation for the sanitary revolution that, by 1875, had stimulated the building of sewers and the provision of clean drinking water in most English cities. It also created an international sanitary hygiene movement that promulgated these new sanitary hygiene ideas, laws, and methods, particularly within the British Empire (Rosen 1958).

In the late nineteenth century, in an atmosphere of heightened health awareness and concern, many medical health officers and other sanitary movement activists became interested in the health implications of a contaminated food supply. The *Lancet* brought the issue to public and professional attention, publishing a series of reports on food adulteration and provoking a parliamentary investigation. These developments occurred just prior to the Bradford incident of 1858, in which 200 people were severely poisoned after eating lozenges. This incident, set against the background of the sanitary revolution and the *Lancet* reports, caused widespread public and professional disquiet and increased the pressure on Parliament to develop food adulteration laws.

Until the 1860s the British food industry had opposed regulation as it had benefited from the state's laissez-faire attitude towards adulteration. With minimal food regulation, manufacturers and retailers could add filler to their products in order to increase weight and volume, and they could also add any quantity of preservative in order to extend shelf life. All of these methods of adulteration could increase profits at both the wholesale level and the retail level.

However, as free trade expanded after 1850, British food manufacturers came under pressure from imported foods. In this new economic climate they realized that laws against adulteration could be used to

keep foreign foods out of their market and to ensure that honest domestic manufacturers and retailers would not be undermined by local
food adulterers (Paulus 1974). For these reasons, by the late 1850s British food manufacturers became increasingly willing to support comprehensive legislation to control food adulteration.

These pressures resulted in the Adulteration of Food and Drink Act,
1860, promulgated within the Department of Inland Revenue, which
made it an offence to knowingly sell adulterated food and which empowered local municipalities to hire food analysts to enforce regulation of the local food supply (French and Phillips 2000). The value of
this legislation was limited because penalties were applied only to illegal retail transactions; the law did not apply to manufacturers and
wholesalers.

While this legislation was largely unenforced, it broke new ground because it was the first consumer protection legislation and the first comprehensive food law to be enacted in the British Empire. It gave official
recognition and support to the role of municipal food analysts and established a fledgling food inspectorate in Britain. Although health activists
helped to force this legislation through Parliament, and although the
legislation was motivated in part by public concerns about food safety,
the act was crafted largely with economic issues in mind (Fallows 1988).

This 1860 British act was strengthened in 1872 when local governments were mandated to appoint properly trained chemists, when food
market inspectors were given powers to seize suspected food samples,
and when manufacturers and wholesalers were made liable for adulterating their products (French and Phillips 2000). The amended British
Adulteration of Food and Drugs Act was passed in 1872 and served as
the template for Canada's Adulteration Act, 1874.

Origins of the Canadian Food Adulteration Legislation
In Canada in the 1860s public concern about adulteration of food and
drink escalated, although the issues were different from those that motivated the British public and legislators. In Canada there were widespread public fears about increases in crime and insanity, which
temperance advocates and many politicians linked to excess drinking
in general and to the drinking of adulterated spirits in particular. Overcrowding in jails and mental institutions was blamed on both intemperance and the consumption of adulterated liquor (Davidson 1949).

In the early 1870s several House and Senate committees were struck to
investigate how intemperance and drinking adulterated liquor affected

criminality. These committees were supported by an active temperance movement led by the Women's Christian Temperance Union, which favoured state-legislated prohibition of alcohol (Valverde 1991). In 1873 temperance advocates presented Parliament with a petition containing 36,000 signatures supporting prohibition (Davidson 1949). Prohibition was opposed by the Roman Catholic Church in Quebec, which viewed it as a potential infringement on the practice of Holy Communion and, therefore, a veiled attack on both the Church and on French Canadians (Curran 1954).

The debates preceding the Food and Drug Act, 1874, were focused on liquor adulteration. The final act, which was placed under the supervision of the Department of Agriculture, was a compromise that appeased the Church by avoiding prohibition and that was at least partially acceptable to temperance advocates because it placed limits on the availability of alcohol. Liquor producers and retailers were required to obtain licences, and an inspection process was established to dissuade manufacturers and retailers from adulterating liquor.

Establishing a System of Food Safety in Canada
Like the public health legislation passed in Ontario (and later adopted by other provinces) around this time (Ostry 1995b, 2006), the 1874 Canadian adulteration legislation was based almost entirely on its British antecedent (Davidson 1949). Although the Adulteration Act was passed due to concerns about alcohol, almost all the early prosecutions that occurred under it dealt with milk and butter. In 1876, 60 percent of the milk sampled under the authority of the act was adulterated, mainly by the addition of chalk and/or water. In 1877 approximately 50 percent of the butter tested was adulterated, although by 1885 this fell to about 19 percent (Davidson 1949).

Over the next quarter of a century legislators amended the Adulteration Act several times and moved its administration from the Department of Agriculture to the Department of Inland Revenue. The amendments resulted in the hiring of a chief analyst, the building of regional laboratories, the expansion of the central laboratory in Ottawa, and improved technical training for all analysts.

Unlike in Britain, in Canada analysts were hired by central rather than municipal governments and were attached either to the central laboratory in Ottawa or to regional laboratories in Ontario, Quebec, the Maritimes, and British Columbia. These analysts were, by and large, poorly trained, badly paid, and empowered to supplement their meagre salaries by charging clients extra fees for their services (Davidson 1949).

This provision was placed in the legislation in order to keep government costs associated with operating the new food inspection service to a minimum. However, the integrity of the system was undermined not only because low wages attracted underqualified analysts but also because the sanctioning of private payments between client and analyst provided fertile ground for corruption and the falsification of results.

Two things were necessary in order to strengthen the system: (1) the establishment of better laboratory techniques and analyst training and (2) the enshrining, in law, of standards for those foods most commonly adulterated. With regard to the latter, the chief analyst in Ottawa was asked to develop positive standards for foods that were commonly adulterated (such as milk). These standards were to define foods in terms of their main chemical constituents. For example, at this time milk was commonly adulterated by the addition of water. Therefore, a definition of milk had to establish a standard for its fat content. Once such a standard was set, it would be possible to declare any deviations from it as adulterated, and it would therefore be possible to launch successful prosecutions whenever this standard was breached.

However, in order to prosecute cases successfully these unofficial food standards had to be established in law. Accordingly, in 1890 the Adulteration Act was amended to enable the government to prescribe standards for food and drugs. The amendment delegated legislative authority to orders-in-council, thereby allowing the government to develop new standards for particular foods without, in each instance, resorting to amending the legislation (Curran 1954).

The 1890 amendment supporting the establishment of positive food standards made Canadian legislation the most advanced in the world. Other countries quickly recognized this Canadian innovation, and within a few years Australia, New Zealand, and South Africa were emulating it (Jukes 1987). The United States was also influenced by the Canadian legislation, incorporating it into the first modern American food adulteration law, the Pure Food Law, 1906 (Curran 1954).

While Canada had established its excellent legislative framework by 1890, it did not, except in the case of milk and a few imported products such as tea, authorize enough money for the analysts to establish positive food standards. This resulted in the system remaining underdeveloped and ineffective.

Canada finally established a number of positive food standards after the passage of the American Pure Food Law, 1906. Passage of this act was motivated almost solely by the scandal resulting from Upton Sinclair's *The Jungle* (Sinclair 1906), which described the Chicago meat-packing industry and stockyards in grim detail, exposing the exploitation of both workers and animals and the incredibly unhygienic standards in the meat processing industry. It also described incidents where workers, who happened to be in the wrong place at the wrong time, ended up as sausage meat. *The Jungle* had a major international impact and, as a shocked public rejected American beef, led to the temporary elimination of imports to Britain and the rest of Europe.

The Pure Food Law, 1906, was the American government's response to this crisis of food safety in the beef industry. The new rules were stringent, and the funding for a new food inspectorate was generous. Very quickly the American system became the international standard.

Immediately upon passage of the Pure Food Law, 1906, the US government established positive food standards. Once published these were adopted, often with little modification, by the Canadian chief analyst and passed into Canadian legislation (Davidson 1949). For example, in 1909 the Canadian chief analyst, with the guidance of an advisory board, used the American legislation as a base to develop standards for a range of dairy products, meats, grains, maple products, and beverages. These were passed in 1911 by an order-in-council but only after being submitted for approval to the Canadian Manufacturers Association (Curran 1954). This indicates that, early in the development of food safety regulation, the Canadian food manufacturing industry was a full partner with the Canadian government in establishing food standards.

In 1907 the federal government passed the Meat and Canned Foods Act. This statute established a regulatory system for all animals intended for slaughter as well as for the inspection of packaged meat products. It also gave the federal government authority to inspect any products prepared for and packed in cans, stipulated labelling requirements for packaged foods, and required that the name of the company, as well as the contents and weight, be marked on the packages. All fish, fruit, and vegetables prepared for export were subject to federal inspection (Canada 1907).

The Meat and Canned Foods Act, 1907, came about for two main reasons: (1) the canning, processing, and mass marketing of foods had become a reality, and (2) this reality was being aided by the rapid concentration of the North American processing industry and the expansion of retail chain stores (Levinstein 1993). The need for an inspection service arose once it became clear that the public was increasingly consuming canned products. The new act increased the workload of the food surveillance system because it expanded the volume, type, and diversity of products for inspection and, for the first time, made inspectors responsible for food labels.

Responsibilities and workload were increased a few years later when the Dairy Industry Act, 1914, was passed to enable the government to more closely monitor the quality of milk, butter, and cheese and to prohibit their being adulterated with water, cream, foreign fat, colour, or preservatives. The act also prohibited the sale and supply of adulterated milk or dairy products to manufacturing plants, bottling plants, or shipping stations, and it allowed the minister of agriculture to specify regulations regarding the classification and branding of dairy products (Canada 1914).

With the Adulteration Act's "teeth" having been sharpened by the 1911 legislative framework for establishing positive food standards, and with the help of the Meat and Canned Foods Act and the Dairy Industry Act, the legal framework for successful adulteration prosecutions was finally in place. However, the civil service was still badly equipped, badly trained, and badly organized, and this seriously hindered successful prosecutions for food contamination. Given its increased responsibilities for the inspection of meat, vegetables, fruit, dairy products, and canned goods, the civil service was strained.

This situation was remedied somewhat in 1913 through an order-in-council establishing new regional laboratories in Halifax, Winnipeg, and Vancouver. In order to speed the pace and quality of analytical work, the laboratories hired properly trained food chemists. By 1919 twenty-five food inspection districts had been established in Canada, and they were staffed with a professionally trained full-time inspectorate (Department of Health Report, 1925).

Thus, by the beginning of the First World War, three main pieces of legislation supervised by the Department of Inland Revenue and the Department of Agriculture formed the backbone of a national food safety, inspection, and surveillance system. The development of properly equipped regional laboratories staffed by well trained food analysts, along with the establishment of a professional inspectorate, had finally produced a fully functioning national system of food inspection.

In 1919 administration of the Adulteration Act was transferred from the Department of Inland Revenue to the Food and Drug Division within the newly formed Department of Health. These institutional and infrastructural developments were enshrined in legislation with the repeal of the Adulteration Act and the passage of the Food and Drug Act, 1920. Transfer of the act to the Department of Health was more than symbolic as it signalled the shift from customs and excise policing of food, and a historical focus on the prevention of economic fraud, towards health surveillance.

The new Department of Health was responsible for coordinating efforts to preserve and improve public health and to conserve child life and promote child welfare – a mandate that gave it jurisdiction over nutritional health issues related to children. This, and the fact that it supervised the Food and Drug Act, gave the health department a strong national role in nutrition policy making both through federal criminal law and through its authority to engage in public health and nutritional health promotion activities.

Under the Food and Drug Act, 1920, food was deemed adulterated if any substance was added to reduce its quality or strength; if any valuable constituent was abstracted from it; if it consisted, in whole or in part, of a diseased animal; if it contained a poisonous ingredient; or if its strength or purity was below standard (Canada 1920).

The new Food and Drug Act also distinguished between adulteration and misbranding (i.e., fraudulent labelling or advertising) of products and provided full salaries for inspectors who had previously been allowed to support themselves by claiming a portion of the penalties they assessed. Twenty-six inspectors were appointed at ports across the country (Vancouver, Halifax, Montreal). While the Food and Drug Act applied to all imports and goods from interprovincial trade, the inspectors focused mainly on imported products (Canada 1920).

Because the nature of fraudulent practices in the food industry began to shift as more foods were sold in packages, as advertising became central to marketing, and as the retail food chain stores proliferated, the new act contained provisions regulating the misbranding of products. The health department was increasingly forced to shift its resources from the inspection, analysis, detection, and prosecution of companies that adulterated their food to fraudulent labelling and/or advertising (see Chapter 6).

Summary

Laws to protect the integrity of the trade in agricultural products and processed food were passed by both French and early British colonial administrations. Modern Canadian food adulteration legislation was passed in 1874. For the first forty-five years this legislation, framed within federal criminal law, focused on the prevention of economic fraud on the part of food wholesalers and retailers. This legislation was adopted, almost verbatim, from British food adulteration legislation that had been passed in 1860.

By 1890 Canada, through a series of amendments, had developed one of the most advanced food adulteration laws in the world; however, due to the undertraining and underfunding of the civil service, it was barely workable. Over the first two decades of the twentieth century – with the adoption of American food standards, increased investment in the food inspectorate, expansion of the central and regional laboratories, and increased salaries for analysts, inspectors, and administrators – the food safety, inspection, and surveillance system began operating effectively nationwide.

The work of the food system began to shift to the inspection and analysis of canned and other processed goods (in order to detect bacterial contamination) as well as to the screening and inspection of labels (in order to detect fraudulent health claims). Public excitement around the discovery of vitamins and manufacturers' growing use of health claims based on the vitamin content of food products increased the burden of the inspectorate and the laboratories.

Moving responsibility for the food safety system from the Department of Inland Revenue to the Department of Health signalled that economic concerns, although still central to the inspectorate, were increasingly being supplanted by new health and health-related nutritional concerns.

The Canadian economy, in the two decades after Confederation, was based mainly on agriculture and resource extraction. After 1880 the pace of industrialization increased, and by 1920 Canada was emerging as an industrial nation. This was not without its problems for the health and nutritional status of the population, and it is to these that I now turn.

2

Infant Mortality, Malnutrition, and Social Reform Prior to the First World War

In the late nineteenth century people began, at first slowly, and by the 1920s more rapidly, to move from the countryside to the cities. As in Britain over half a century earlier, so in Canada the influx of people into cities, whose basic public health infrastructure was inadequate, led to increased urban mortality rates due largely to infectious diseases (Ostry 1995a, 1995b).

The most vulnerable at this time of transition were infants, particularly those who were raised in poverty and artificially fed. And the most vulnerable of the vulnerable were the babies of working and impoverished women who were undernourished or malnourished. As Canada industrialized social reformers began to agitate more strongly for the federal government to tackle problems of malnutrition, particularly among poor urban women and their infants.

This chapter explains the growth in concern over malnutrition and its relationship to infant mortality. The crisis over infant mortality drove the social and health reform movements in the late nineteenth and early twentieth centuries, and this, in turn, pushed the federal government to play a stronger role in national nutrition and health policy at the end of the First World War. As well, the twin issues of malnutrition and infant mortality shaped the scope, direction, and tenor of the first nutritional education programs, which the federal government developed in the 1920s.

The first section of this chapter describes the nutritional status of Canadians in the late nineteenth century. Although data are limited and based only on studies conducted in Toronto and Montreal, they do allow for some tentative conclusions. The second section provides a description of the changing nutritional status of the Canadian population from the beginning of the twentieth century to the end of the First World War. The final section describes the social and political changes that followed the First World War and that led the federal government to adopt a nutritional policy-making role.

The Nutritional Status of Canadians in the Late Nineteenth Century

At Confederation approximately one-quarter of the Canadian population lived in cities and towns; however, by 1900 over 40 percent lived in urban centres. Toronto and Montreal were the largest Canadian cities, and by 1900 they were responsible for 60 percent of the nation's manufacturing activity. The last quarter of the nineteenth century was a difficult one for many city and town dwellers because: (1) a major economic depression occurred in 1875, lasted for a decade, and was followed by sluggish economic growth until 1896; (2) the pace of immigration to urban centres, both from abroad and from the countryside, depressed the price of unskilled labour; (3) the pace of industrialization increased; and (4) these changes took place prior to the establishment of many basic health, welfare, and labour laws and institutions, with the result that they tended to lower the standard of living of the urban poor, particularly women and children (Ward and Ward 1984). As well, in the last quarter of the nineteenth century urban workers were almost entirely dependent on the cash economy for their ability to purchase food. Urbanization resulted in people being separated from the land, and the lack of garden space, particularly in Montreal and Toronto, made it difficult to grow food.

An indication of the declining nutritional status of poor women is shown in a study of infant birth weights at Montreal's University Lying-In Hospital (where approximately 2 percent of the city's children were born) between 1851 to 1905 (Ward and Ward 1984). During this fifty-four-year period the mean weight of infants born at the hospital fell steadily by 430 grams (11.9 percent). This evidence suggests "serious malnutrition as the primary cause of birth-weight decline" as "the quality of diet among poor women in the city seems to have deteriorated badly, particularly after 1880" (Ward and Ward 1984, 337).

With industrialization, particularly in Montreal and Toronto, came increasing female and child employment. For example, by 1871 women and children comprised 42 percent of the industrial workforce in Montreal (Ames 1972) and 34 percent in Toronto (Kealey 1980). Although a number of provincial statutes were enacted after 1884 to increase worker protection through Workers' Compensation and to reduce the length of the work week, these excluded the "single largest category of employed women, domestics" (Ursel 1992, 94). And, while factory work, which in 1880s Ontario employed approximately one-third of female workers, paid subsistence wages, it did so only if women workers maintained a fifty-four-hour week (Ursel 1992).

These limited data indicate that, at least in Toronto and Montreal, the Canadian industrial revolution in the last quarter of the nineteenth century may have adversely affected the economic position and nutritional status of poor urban women and their children. While these data provide some indication of the prevalence of undernutrition in Montreal and Toronto, virtually nothing is known of the nutritional status of people living in other regions of Canada during the last half of the nineteenth century.

Improvement in Nutritional Status to the 1920s

While the last quarter of the nineteenth century may have been a difficult time for the urban poor, it is likely that nutritional status had begun to improve by the turn of the twentieth century as twenty-five years of depression and economic stagnation ended in 1896 and a period of rising incomes, which lasted until the First World War, got under way. Increasing incomes may have improved access to food, at least for some of the urban poor. As well as economic growth, the era from 1884 (beginning with the passage of Ontario's Factory Act) to 1914 saw the promulgation of many of Canada's basic welfare and public health statutes, such as workers' compensation legislation and municipal sanitation legislation, including (at least in some Canadian cities) legislation to improve the quality and cleanliness of milk and meat supplies, all of which likely contributed to improvements in the health and nutritional status of the poor (Ostry 2006).

As well, the analysis of several studies of children's growth rates in Toronto between 1891 and 1974 demonstrate that a long and sustained upward movement in these rates began in the 1890s (as in many North American cities) and was probably due to a combination of higher incomes, the beginnings of a social safety net, and better sanitary conditions, housing, and nutrition (Hoppa and Garlie 1998). Studies in Britain over the same time period demonstrate links between increasing working-class income, urban public health improvements, improved nutritional status, and improved child growth rates. It is likely that the increases in growth observed in the Toronto study (beginning in the 1890s) were also due to a complex combination of these factors (Floud et al. 1990). These data cannot be reliably extrapolated to other Canadian cities as Toronto was ahead of them in developing a public health and sanitary infrastructure, including a municipal milk and food inspection system. In other words, the growth rates among children observed in this study may have been unique to Toronto (MacDougall 1990).

It is clear that the leading medical health officers of the day, particularly those based in Toronto, were concerned about sanitary hygiene, municipal development, poverty, and hunger – particularly among Canada's urban women and children (MacDougall 1990) – and that social activists (church, labour, and women's groups) were highly mobilized around these issues throughout the late nineteenth century and the early twentieth century (Ursel 1992; Valverde 1991).

In spite of considerable agitation for social and public health reform, the first medical investigations of undernutrition and malnutrition in Canada were not conducted until the end of the First World War. The First World War heightened concerns about malnutrition in Canada in part because of the rapid increases in the price of food, which began in the middle of the war and continued into the early 1920s (Britnell and Fowke 1962). The military was also worried as "in the examination of recruits so many men were found to be unfit for military service as a result of conditions following malnutrition that attention was then brought to bear on the condition as it appeared in children" (Brown and Davis 1921, 66). Thus wartime concerns about military fitness among young males in Canada (which were echoed in many other nations at this time and which, for the first time – except in Britain, where these same issues had been raised during the Boer War – made nutrition a national security issue) led to two investigations of malnutrition among Toronto schoolchildren.

An investigation of 2,843 elementary school children, enrolled in four schools, was conducted in conjunction with the Toronto Department of Public Health. It showed that "44 percent were 7 percent or more underweight and 751 or 26 percent were 10-12 percent underweight" (Brown and Davis 1921, 69). By extrapolating these results to the entire Toronto elementary school population, the authors estimated that 26 percent of Toronto students were undernourished "and in a serious state of health" (Brown and Davis 1921, 69). This study also concluded that malnutrition was found equally among high- and low-income students.

A second study, conducted in 1921 and focusing on 370 children who attended the Nutritional Clinic at Toronto's Hospital for Sick Children, found that malnutrition "was just as prevalent with the rich as with the poor" and that malnutrition cases were to be found in equal proportion among breastfed and bottle-fed babies (Macdougall 1925, 26). According to the investigator, the cause of malnutrition in approximately half these cases involved mismanagement and lack of discipline in the home.

In particular, "the first evidence of lack of home control is the fact that the child nurses 15 to 18 months. When the parent fails to control a child of that age, what success need one expect in dealing with this same child at 10 years of age?" (MacDougall 1925, 28). The author attributed only forty-four of the 370 (12 percent) cases of malnutrition to "improper diet and faulty food habits."

Both these studies of Toronto schoolchildren show that, just after the First World War, in spite of likely improvements in nutritional status since the turn of the century, undernutrition or malnutrition (never accurately defined) was a problem for many of the city's poor children. The authors of both these (not very well designed) studies claimed that there were no differences in nutritional status across income levels, and they were quick to blame mothers' "lack of discipline" for the undernourishment of their children. The timing of these studies (during the years immediately following the First World War) may have produced results that were somewhat atypical for the first two decades of the twentieth century. It must also be remembered that they were conducted during years of extreme inflation in Canadian food prices.

It is possible that the nutritional status of the rural population during the industrial transformation of the late nineteenth century was better than was the nutritional status of urban populations. This is because, among rural families, lack of income did not block access to food to the same extent as it did among urban families. And, as has been seen in other countries in the midst of industrial revolutions, urban populations bear the brunt of the inadequacies of public health infrastructure as cities slowly develop sewers, garbage disposal, clean water, and food inspection services. Thus general living and nutritional conditions in the cities were likely less healthy than were those in the countryside. These differences between rural and urban regions are illustrated by Ontario's mortality statistics, which indicate that, in 1905, as the industrial transition was maturing, mortality rates among children in urban areas (a very sensitive indicator of living and nutritional conditions) were approximately 35 percent greater than they were in rural parts of the province (Ursel 1992).

Infant Mortality and Social Reform

In the late nineteenth century infant mortality rates in Canada were among the highest in the Western world (Comacchio 1993). And in the province of Quebec in the first decade of the twentieth century the infant mortality rate was 146.4 per 1,000 live births – approximately one-third higher than in the rest of Canada (Bernier 1989).

Until the 1940s Montreal and Quebec City were two of the most un-healthy cities in North America, let alone in Canada. According to a 1901 survey 40 percent of deaths in the city of Quebec from 1891 to 1900 were caused by infectious disease. Densely populated areas were more affected, and young children were especially susceptible. In Mon-treal between 1893 and 1895 children accounted for half of all deaths (Bernier 1989).

The industrial revolution and concomitant social upheavals that were under way in Canada in the 1880s and 1890s provoked increasing pres-sure for social reform, in particular the alleviation of poverty, which was seen as the root cause of high infant mortality. In English Canada the reform movement was largely spearheaded by alliances between the Protestant Church, welfare organizations, and the new and rapidly grow-ing Canadian trade union movement. Between 1890 and 1914 a number of organizations, such as the National Council of Women, the Women's Christian Temperance Union, and the Social Service Council of Canada, were formed largely to provide education and charity for the poor and to encourage the government to take a more active role in providing social welfare, particularly for children (Allen 1971; Moscovitch and Drover 1987; Valverde 1991).

This widespread social reform movement fused Christian piety with the socialist activism of the growing trade union movement. Much of this activism was focused on traditionally female spheres of concern, such as prohibition of alcohol, family and child health and welfare is-sues, and female suffrage, which gained increasing momentum in the decade prior to the First World War. This "social gospel" phenomenon, "which was not a uniquely Canadian movement, but was part of a wide-spread attempt in Europe and North America to revive and develop Christian social insights and to apply them to the emerging forms of collective society," was the ideology that united disparate activist or-ganizations and that, by the end of the First World War, pressed the state to address social welfare issues (including malnutrition among women and children) in order to reduce high rates of infant mortality (Allen 1971, 2).

In the first decades of the twentieth century numerous groups were involved in the war against infant mortality. In Quebec Les Cercles des Fermières and a variety of other women's organizations provided much of the force behind early maternal and child welfare campaigns (Arnup 1994). The National Council of Women of Canada established the Vic-torian Order of Nurses in 1897, which visited mothers in their homes and provided instruction in infant care and feeding. And, across Canada, women's institutes played an important role in child welfare work, especially in rural areas, by establishing health services, providing school lunches, and distributing health literature.

Just before the First World War Dr. Helen MacMurchy (1910, 1911, 1912), a Toronto physician specializing in child care, obstetrics, and gynecology, authored three reports on infant mortality in Ontario. She attributed high infant mortality to poverty and unsanitary living conditions. Although MacMurchy recognized the relationship between poverty and malnutrition and ill health, she did not recommend economic reforms; rather, she focused on education, particularly the promotion of breastfeeding. According to MacMurchy and many other social and public health reformers, high infant mortality would be solved through educating mothers in proper methods of child rearing and infant feeding rather than through structural and political reform.

Prior to the First World War the campaign to address infant mortality in both rural and urban areas was uncoordinated and disorganized. Boards of health existed at the provincial level and in most urban centres, but Canadians living in rural areas had limited access to medical services and health care facilities. Voluntary groups, while important, were not able to meet the huge need for child welfare work. Many groups pushed the federal government to tackle infant mortality.

In the decade prior to the First World War pressure built to create a federal children's bureau. In 1912 a children's bureau was established in the United States, within the Department of Labour (Rosen 1958; Schnell 1987). In 1913 the newly formed Social Service Council of Canada (SSCC), mainly a coalition of activist church organizations, held a congress in which a resolution was passed urging the federal government to follow the American lead.

The First World War, with its large loss of life, had traumatized the nation and highlighted the fact that a strong, vibrant population was essential to national security. "We are only now discovering that Empires and States are built up of babies. Cities are dependent for their continuance on babies. Armies are recruited only if and when we have cared for our babies" (Arnup 1994, 21). The health of children was increasingly seen as the key to achieving national goals. And, with the public health reforms that occurred in some Canadian cities during the previous decades, governments, including the federal government, realized that infant deaths were preventable.

The primary reason for the creation of the federal Department of Health in 1919 was to provide medical care and rehabilitation services to returning soldiers (Ostry 1994, 1995a, 1995b). At that time, while important, child welfare was a lesser consideration. However, due to intense lobbying by the SSCC and affiliated organizations, and due to the fact that women had just obtained the right to vote, many in government felt that the establishment of a division of child welfare would meet the concerns of these organizations and, at the same time, help to secure the votes of newly enfranchised Canadian women (Schnell 1987).

The Division of Child Welfare was formed in 1919, and Helen MacMurchy was immediately appointed as its director. In 1921 the division helped establish the National Council on Child Welfare. This council played a major role in coordinating women's and medical organizations and government departments with regard to child welfare work, and it ensured that linkages were maintained between these organizations and the Division of Child Welfare. Through its publication, *The Canadian Mother's Book*, the Division of Child Welfare produced the first national nutrition education program directed at expectant and new mothers and their infants (see Chapter 5). At the same time as the Child Welfare Division was becoming involved in nutrition education, the Department of Agriculture began a campaign to market foods. Like the former, the latter also targeted women and children.

Summary

Infant mortality rates in Canada were extremely high in the nineteenth and early twentieth centuries. And rates in the province of Quebec during this time were approximately one-third higher than they were in the rest of the country.

Limited data on infant mortality in Montreal indicate that, at least for the poor, rates deteriorated during the period of intense industrialization in the last quarter of the nineteenth century. This was likely due to the rapid influx of people into cities that had limited public health infrastructure and the conditions of which disempowered the working and destitute poor. As well, the last quarter of the nineteenth century experienced a prolonged economic downturn, which ended only in 1896.

After the 1890s several long-term growth studies in Toronto and Montreal indicated that the nutritional status of urban Canadians may have begun to improve, as it had in many other North American cities at this time. These data are sparse, are only available for Toronto and Montreal, and cannot be readily extrapolated to other regions of Canada.

While concern mounted over infant mortality, the first investigations of the relationship between infant mortality and malnutrition were not conducted until the end of the First World War. These studies measured the weight of Toronto's schoolchildren and concluded that undernutrition was fairly widespread among poor children. Because these studies were conducted during the years when food price inflation was at a historic high, it is not clear to what extent they reflect the levels of undernutrition since the turn of the century or to what extent they can be extrapolated to other Canadian cities (let alone rural regions).

By the end of the first decade of the twentieth century women's struggle to obtain the vote increased, as did child welfare advocates' and public health reformers' agitation for the establishment of a federal Department of Health and an active division of child welfare that was focused on child health. The pressure from these reformers, in conjunction with the new political and social conditions following the First World War, led to the formation of a department of health and a division of child welfare headed by Helen MacMurchy.

The new Division of Child Welfare developed and disseminated nutrition advice to expectant and new mothers, marking the federal government's first foray into nutrition education. The establishment of the division was the culmination of forty years of activism on the part of women, the church, trade unionists, and professionals who found common cause (often under the banner of the social gospel) campaigning for women's suffrage, the reduction of poverty, the improvement of working conditions, and the institution of social and urban reform.

Chapter 3 discusses the medical profession and infant feeding to the 1920s. In the mid-nineteenth century the medical profession played only a marginal role in advising mothers on infant feeding; however, by the turn of the twentieth century physicians were involved in dispensing advice to mothers and, increasingly, to governments, particularly regarding the nutrition of infants.

3

The Medical Profession and Infant Feeding to the 1920s

While the federal government, which was at first motivated by economic and criminal concerns, developed the food safety system, the medical profession in North America slowly built its organization and its reputation with the public and, in the process, became an important disseminator of advice on nutrition.

In Canada the medical profession began organizing in the years following Confederation (Ostry 2006). In the mid-nineteenth century physicians did not enjoy the high social, professional, and economic status that they do today. They relied heavily on purging and bleeding treatments, which were ineffective, painful, and invasive. As, by the 1870s, physicians were only slowly beginning to accept Joseph Lister's new anti-septic methods, surgery was usually fatal. Anaesthesia was crude and ineffective, and surgical techniques and instruments were similarly inadequate (Roland 1981). Throughout the nineteenth century the public frequented not only physicians but also homeopaths, naturopaths, and illegal practitioners of all kinds (Heagerty 1928).

This changed in the 1880s, following the discovery that germs caused disease, and in the 1890s, following dramatic advances in surgery, obstetrics, and gynecology, and the development of effective treatments for fairly common infectious diseases such as diphtheria (1894) (Shortt 1981). By the turn of the century physicians possessed accurate pathological information about the diseases that they treated, reasonable physiological knowledge upon which to base their treatments, and diagnostic tools backed by an increasingly sophisticated public health and hospital infrastructure (Ostry 1995a, 1995b; Shortt 1981). And by 1910 medical education had been reformed and placed on a scientific footing – an occurrence that vastly improved the quality of Canadian medical graduates (Flexner 1910).

As the medical profession became more organized and effective its status increased. Physicians were increasingly respected care givers and advisors. And governments, particularly after the turn of the century when they began to take responsibility for the health of their populations, began to rely on the medical profession for scientific and medical expertise and policy direction.

The last half of the nineteenth century also witnessed the invention of artificial infant foods, their widespread promotion and marketing, and the beginning of a long decline in breastfeeding, which was not arrested until the late 1970s (Myres 1979, 1981). This era also saw the birth and expansion of pediatrics, which was due almost entirely to its promotion of artificial infant feeding, particularly among its fee-paying middle- and upper-class patients.

While many pediatricians and other physicians promoted artificial infant feeding, others, alarmed by the clear links between this type of feeding and infant mortality, were strongly opposed to it. Alliances between those in the medical profession opposed to artificial infant feeding and child welfare and public health reformers grew after the turn of the century.

This chapter outlines the involvement of the medical profession, particularly pediatricians, in artificial infant feeding prior to 1919. It begins with a discussion of the late-nineteenth-century shift in child rearing philosophy and practices as mothers were inundated with scientific and expert advice about child rearing. The second section outlines the role of pediatrics in this shift and its rise in relation to infant feeding. The third section looks at pediatrics in Canada up to the end of the First World War and assesses the profession's ambiguous role both in providing expertise on infant feeding and in promoting breastfeeding. At this time, milk depots and child welfare clinics were established in many Canadian cities. The fourth section looks at how, in attending these clinics, poor women gained access to physicians and pediatricians and received advice on infant feeding. The last section looks at how upper- and middle-class women gained access to these professionals through paying fees for their services. It was during this era that rates of breastfeeding began to decline, especially and most quickly among wealthy, well educated women.

Scientific Motherhood

During the late nineteenth century, science was equated with rational reform, and professors, physicians, and social workers gained greater social status and responsibility. Many physicians were able to bridge the rational and scientific world with the social roles of the reformer. By the second decade of the twentieth century, as governments expanded their role in social and health policy, the medical profession was called upon to interpret and apply new scientific knowledge by accepting roles as health inspectors, directors of public health clinics, and medical officers.

The beginning of the twentieth century also saw a dramatic shift in ideas about child rearing. Just as industry benefited from the application of scientific knowledge, so, too, did the household. The general population's growing respect for science-based technology enhanced women's acceptance of new ideas of scientific household management and child rearing. The new scientific motherhood was based on "the insistence that women require expert scientific and medical advice to raise their children healthfully" (Apple 1995). Motherhood was viewed as too important, particularly at a time when concerns about persistently high rates of infant mortality dominated child welfare and health departments, to be left to love, instinct, and nature.

Pediatricians and Infant Feeding

Until the middle of the nineteenth century maternal breastfeeding or wet-nursing was the sole method of infant feeding. When breast milk was not available a variety of substitutes were used to feed babies; however, due to generally unsanitary conditions, infants usually failed to thrive and often died.

By the middle of the nineteenth century, as a by-product of advances in chemistry and nutritional sciences, artificial infant foods had been invented. These artificial foods were extremely dangerous for three reasons. First, they were usually made from dried cow's milk combined with starch or malt, desiccated malt extract, or a cereal base, and they were usually reconstituted by the addition of cow's milk or water. Given that, for many Canadians living in both rural and urban areas, clean water and disease-free pasteurized or certified milk were not available, the addition of either of these non-sterile liquids increased the risk of passing disease-causing bacteria to the infant. Second, at this time vitamins were not added to commercially manufactured artificial foods, with the result that reliance on these "dead foods" usually led to vitamin deficiency diseases in infants (particularly scurvy and rickets). And third, because the carbohydrate content of artificial foods was often too high, babies who consumed them were often too fat and suffered from "severe gastro-intestinal upset" (Spohn 1920).

The medical profession's attitude towards artificial foods was mixed. In the United States many pediatricians were involved in the manufacture and sale of artificial infant foods. However, the rise of mass-produced commercially prepared artificial foods threatened those pediatric specialist who preferred to sell their skills directly to paying patients. Pediatricians involved in this latter type of medical practice stressed the need for carefully tailored, individually designed artificial infant foods. Their suspicion of commercially produced artificial foods is encapsulated by Rorke (1916, 68): "The usual patent foods on the market are unsuitable and undesirable from the pediatrician's point of view. All of them are put up for any child and, therefore, make no allowance for the particular digestive ability of the individual infant."

Still other pediatricians felt strongly that babies should only be breastfed. And others, who were often faced with poor, overworked women who were not able to breastfeed because of the pressures of their home and work conditions, attempted to make pasteurized or certified milk available, along with instructions on "clean" artificial feeding.

As clean water and milk became more widely available, and as artificial food manufacturers began to add vitamins to their infant formulas, physicians' attitudes towards artificial feeding became more favourable. From the 1880s to the 1920s cow's milk was increasingly preferred to commercial artificial infant food. This was because physicians saw that children raised on clean cow's milk did better than children fed with artificial foods. In retrospect, it is clear that this was due to the presence of vitamins in the former and the lack of vitamins in the latter. Increasingly, prior to the discovery of vitamins, professionals came to believe that cow's milk contained some unknown elements that were essential to nourishing an infant (Rudolf 1912). However, in cow's milk these elements were present in different proportions than they were in human milk.

With the shift towards cow's milk, various schools of infant feeding developed, all of which had the goal of modifying cow's milk by diluting it or adding to it so that it would resemble human milk. The use of the "percentage method" required close surveillance of the infant. Different dilutions of cow's milk were prescribed according to the age of the infant and were altered during illness (after an analysis of the child's stools). Infants differed in their digestive ability and nutritional needs; hence, a variation of even 0.1 percent in a given ingredient was believed to make the difference between an ill-fed baby and a well-fed one.

The percentage method was just one of several competing methods of infant feeding. Physicians who desired to learn this complex art devoted themselves to several years of study at the appropriate schools. Pediatrics soon made infant feeding central to its practice. Many pediatricians focused exclusively on developing and prescribing infant formulas.

Views on the appropriate content of infant food would change rapidly, and often completely reverse themselves, over a short period. In 1924 Goldbloom (1924, 710) mused that "the pendulum has swung. Ten years ago we were adding alkalis to milk as the only and proper way to feed infants ... Now we are adding acid to milk in order to neutralize buffer substances." Similarly, Rudolf (1912) commented that "infant feeding theory has run riot" and that "the proteins, the fat, and the sugar of cow's milk have each in turn been blamed" for digestion difficulties in infants.

Methods of mixing, and formulas for modifying, cow's milk varied considerably from physician to physician. Although most used a combination of milk, water, and sugar, the exact proportions and additions were determined by individual physicians after examining infants' stools. In a process called "divination by stool" and "coprophyllic fetishism," physicians would determine the cause of an infant's ills and modify its formula accordingly (Goldbloom 1945).

Pediatrics and Artificial Feeding in Canada
At a meeting of the Pediatric Section of the Toronto Academy of Medicine, Robert Rudolf (1912), a professor at the University of Toronto, commented that "percentage feeding is chiefly of American growth." This may have been because, at this time in Canada, pediatrics was relatively underdeveloped (MacGregor 1923). Although pediatrics had established itself in Britain and the United States at the end of the nineteenth century, Canada lagged behind. In 1914 there were two pediatricians in Canada (Commachio 1993). By 1922 the Society for the Study of the Diseases of Children had been established. Although few in number, Canadian pediatricians took on an increasingly important role in child welfare in general and in the development of scientific principles for rearing children, for preparing infant formula, and for scheduling infant feeding (Brown 1919). These services were initially provided to a small group of paying middle-class patients who were interested in using scientific knowledge to improve the health of their families and children.

In Canada the Department of Pediatrics at the University of Toronto was the centre for the study of infant feeding. Allan Brown, the head of the department, emphasized the need for systematic child training. It was believed that, through education and the application of sound scientific principles, parents could successfully raise their children.

One of the keys to scientific child rearing was the establishment of fixed times for every activity. Children were to be fed at regular intervals – even if this meant waking the child.

Brown (1933, 266) describes the role of the physician in determining an infant's needs as follows: "If a baby is not thriving, it is either because there is something wrong with the infant or the food is deficient in some way; and it is up to the physician to determine the cause." The field of infant feeding was deemed to be extremely complex, and mothers were increasingly told that they did not have the knowledge and skills to determine what was best for their babies. According to Brown, when determining the best artificial formula for an infant, one had to contend with "the popular delusion [that] their adaptation to the physiologic needs of each infant is so simple that the process can be safely entrusted to little mothers."

By the mid-1920s, pediatricians were increasingly acting as consultants to public health departments and other government agencies, and they provided advice to mothers in magazines, newspapers, books, radio, and health publications. They were also connected with major children's hospitals, child welfare clinics, health departments, and medical schools, where they were engaged in research and were heavily involved in teaching general practitioners and young pediatricians (Commachio 1993).

The application of principles of scientific management to child rearing led to the increased prominence and authority of physicians in child care and signified a move away from tradition-bound mothering. Although mothers assumed ultimate responsibility for the health of their families, they were encouraged to frequently consult experts for advice. Through educating mothers in the area of infant feeding, physicians believed they would be able to significantly reduce the high rates of child mortality.

While middle- and upper-class women had access to physicians and pediatricians, some poor women were also able to have such access through public hospitals and the child welfare clinics (which were popping up in many Canadian cities just before and during the First World War). Increasingly, these became sites for disseminating nutritional information to poor women and their babies.

Child Welfare Clinics, Breastfeeding, and Artificial Feeding

At the turn of the century child welfare advocates in Britain established a number of "pure milk" depots in poor urban neighbourhoods. These supplied working-class mothers with clean cow's milk (either certified or pasteurized) and, at the same time, actively promoted breastfeeding. Over time, these evolved into perinatal clinics with a home visiting component. In Canada this system, which entailed having a supervisory clinic located in poor areas coupled with perinatal home visits, became the model for most child welfare work during the first half of the twentieth century (Comacchio 1993). Like those established in British cities, the child welfare clinics established in Toronto, Hamilton, Ottawa, and London prior to the First World War began as pure milk depots; however, by war's end they had evolved into more broadly focused child welfare clinics and were providing instruction to mothers of young children.

The Babies' Dispensary Guild was established in 1911 in Hamilton. Building upon the milk-depot model, the guild initially encouraged women to bring their babies to be examined by the physician. Over time, the guild shifted to a focus on education and information. Babies were examined and breastfeeding or certified milk recommended (Arnup 1994). By 1913 milk depots were becoming "more and more a school for the mother instead of merely a depot to sell milk, as most of the milk that comes to the city is good and we encourage the mothers to nurse their babies and drink the milk themselves" (Commachio 1993, 50).

Little mothers' leagues were another source of scientific information on infant feeding and child rearing. In Manitoba, beginning in 1912, public health nurses formed numerous little mothers' leagues. In 1917 the first little mothers' leagues were organized in Vancouver (Breeze 1926). These classes targeted girls in Grade 8 and provided instruction on personal hygiene, care of infants and children, home nursing, and first aid. Girls were told that mother's milk was the safest and best food for the first nine months of an infant's life, and they were provided with information on why condensed milk and artificial foods should rarely be used. After nine months babies were to be weaned and fruit juices were to be added to their diet (Wells 1926).

During the early part of the twentieth century the extensive educational efforts of various voluntary and governmental agencies in child welfare clinics and in milk depots in working-class neighbourhoods were believed to have resulted in increased rates of breastfeeding: "Wherever propaganda for more breast feeding has been instituted there has occurred a marked improvement. In 1917, in Toronto, such a campaign was instituted in the various child welfare clinics ... so that even with the improvement in the technique of artificial feeding, breast feeding is more prevalent throughout our clinics than it was twelve years ago" (Brown 1931, 518).

Dr. A. Chandler (1929), medical director of the Montreal Child Welfare Association, also believed that breastfeeding rates had increased from 1900 to 1920, but he, along with other Canadian experts, realized that, after 1920, a serious decline in breastfeeding had set in. This was attributed to numerous factors: maternal ignorance, advertising campaigns that exaggerated the benefits of artificial infant foods, physician indifference to (and ignorance of) breastfeeding, fast-paced modern living, and the employment of mothers outside the home. Chandler and others also blamed poverty – specifically, crowded apartment dwellings, conditions leading to "mental stress," minimum food allowances, inadequate housing and heating, and lack of proper clothing (Canadian Council on Child Welfare 1930; Chandler 1929).

Chandler also suggested that the growth of child welfare clinics, and particularly the practice of weighing babies (which was common in these clinics), paradoxically contributed to the decline in breastfeeding after 1920. At each visit to the health centre infants were weighed and measured, and mothers knew that their children should be gaining weight regularly. However, breastfeeding mothers were also able to compare their infants with those who were artificially fed. As the latter tended to gain weight more quickly than did breastfed babies, Chandler believed that the high weaning rates among breastfeeding mothers was due to their being discouraged by the growth rates of their babies.

Chandler also became increasingly concerned about the role of physicians in the decline of breastfeeding. "When the obstetrician hands the baby over to the pediatrist, does he not imply that he is not familiar with modern methods of artificial feeding rather than not being conversant with breast feeding?" (Chandler 1929, 263) He also commented on competition between pediatricians, which often resulted in "show[ing] off our skill in artificial feeding rather than keeping a baby on the breast, which is less spectacular and much more difficult" (ibid.).

By the late 1920s physicians working in clinics in poor neighbourhoods began to realize that it was necessary to separate mothers who were breastfeeding from those who were feeding their babies cow's milk and formula as, when these two practices were taught side by side, artificial feeding tended to undermine breastfeeding (see Chapter 6). While breastfeeding was on the decline among poor women, by the 1920s it was plummeting among the upper classes.

Breastfeeding and Artificial Feeding among the Well-To-Do

Commenting on a 1917 survey on breastfeeding in Toronto, Brown (1933, 266) noted that "the well-to-do of Toronto and environs nursed their infants less often than did the members of the poorer classes." The increase in popularity of artificial feeding among the middle and upper classes was not entirely puzzling. Many problems with artificial feeding – such as exposure to contaminated milk, improper methods of feeding, bad surroundings, heat, humidity, dirt, and overcrowding – had declined since the turn of the century in many Canadian cities and were not major concerns for people with education and income. The increasing availability of refrigeration and pasteurized milk, and easier methods of sterilizing equipment, meant that artificial feeding was not as dangerous as it had been in the past – at least for those with good incomes.

At this time, artificial infant foods were relatively expensive (Spohn 1920). The compelling advertisements from the infant formula industry, which produced and disseminated information about the virtues of artificial feeding, were clearly directed at those who could afford them. According to Brown (1933, 267), one of the reasons that well-to-do women abandoned breastfeeding was because they "receive[d] the full onslaught of a whirlwind of advertisements and of propaganda most ingeniously worded to assail their faith." He also observed that, among the upper classes, successful nursing no longer seemed to be a matter of prestige. In the past the inability to breastfeed had been viewed as a woman's personal failure to fulfill her "natural" duties as a mother; now women seemed indifferent to their inability to breastfeed.

With the increased respect for scientific methods of child rearing among the upper classes the idea that a woman had to breastfeed if she were to fulfill her maternal duties had begun to shift. As Brown (1933, 267) commented: "Many who would have breastfed have not dared persevere under the implication that this is an ordinary way of infant nurture, and that babies must not be deprived of anything 'scientific' or 'good' merely to save the instinct of the mother to nourish and care for them herself. Fathers anxious that their wives should be comfortable are readily persuaded of the 'strain' of breastfeeding." And, as he noted further, this led to an undermining of breastfeeding as mothers began "to believe that they 'can't nurse their babies' or that the offspring of their efforts will be 'bonnier' if not subjected to the toils of the breast" (ibid.).

Summary

In the late nineteenth century the medical profession and child welfare experts developed scientific methods both for rearing and feeding children. The supplanting of "natural" with scientific approaches to living first occurred among the upper classes. While the wealthy and educated were the first to take up these ideas, the middle classes and the poor were not far behind.

The rise of pediatrics mirrored the rise of the medical profession. Particularly in the United States, many in the new specialty developed and marketed artificial infant foods in the era before vitamins were discovered. Without vitamins and served alone (and/or diluted with unclean water or cow's milk) these foods were a virtual death warrant for many infants. As conditions of sanitation and hygiene in urban regions improved, the risks from unclean water and cow's milk declined, although the dangers of feeding an infant only artificial foods remained until vitamins were discovered in the 1920s and added to artificial foods.

The popularity of pediatrics grew hand-in-hand with the popularity of artificial infant feeding. Infant feeding was particularly promoted more among patients with high income because both pediatricians and infant foods were expensive.

Many pediatricians were skeptical of commercially produced infant foods either because such foods enabled patients to by-pass their services or because they believed that breastfeeding was best. Those not involved in the commercial infant food industry increasingly marketed their services by arguing that each infant had precise and complicated feeding needs (which of course needed constant adjustment) that required their expert attention.

In the era prior to the discovery of vitamins (roughly from 1875 to the First World War), when the deadly nature of artificial infant foods became clear, many physicians and pediatricians advised their patients to use cow's milk (variously diluted) and offered their services as experts who could appropriately modify this often unclean liquid. The birth of the percentage method (along with other complex methods) of feeding infants cow's milk, bolstered by divination rituals involving infant stools, also helped to consolidate the role of pediatricians as nutritional advisors.

While in Canada pediatrics did not evolve as quickly or as early as it did in the United States and Britain, in the 1920s the new specialty increasingly began to advise governments, public institutions, and patients. More and more often, as child welfare clinics and milk depots became established, the artificial feeding methods utilized by upper-class women were also being used by working-class women.

The advice dispensed in child welfare clinics was often contradictory. Differing advice about artificial feeding and breastfeeding was an expression of scientific and pseudo-scientific conflicts within the medical profession as well as of conflicts between physicians and the increasingly vocal child welfare activists. Advice promoting breastfeeding among poor working women was often ineffective.

As Chandler and other experts began to note in the mid-1920s, the juxtaposition of breastfed and artificially fed babies in child welfare clinics, particularly with regard to the highly visible act of weighing babies, appeared to weaken the appeal of breastfeeding among poor women. It is not clear whether the move to artificial feeding among poor women was driven by work pressures or by the fact that safe and clean cow's milk was often available at these clinics and increasingly in some cities through the general milk supply. Whatever the reason, the trend to more artificial feeding in working and poor women was likely reinforced by the even more rapid abandonment of breastfeeding by wealthier and better educated women.

Women's move away from breastfeeding in the 1920s was the beginning of a long decline, which only ended in the early 1970s. This decline in breastfeeding was not unique to Canada but, rather, occurred at the same time in most other industrial nations.

As artificial feeding became more firmly entrenched in the 1920s, government nutrition experts and medical and non-medical reformers moved to aggressively promote breastfeeding. While public health officials and reformers promoted breastfeeding, particularly following the discovery of vitamins, many physicians advised their patients to feed their infants cow's milk and/or artificial infant foods. As Canadian dairy herds and milk became less diseased, it was increasingly possible to feed cow's milk to infants with relative safety. Accordingly, in the 1920s the historical image of cow's milk as a dangerous and contaminated substance began to change. These developments are outlined in Chapter 4.

4
Cow's Milk: A New Image for the 1920s

While the federal government had, by the mid-1920s, established an efficient and effective system of food inspection supported by well equipped laboratories and a well trained inspectorate (see Chapter 1), cow's milk, an increasingly important food for children, was often unpasteurized, contaminated, and obtained from tuberculosis-infested cattle. Obviously, this posed a danger to the health of children. Most public health legislation, which is under provincial jurisdiction, empowers municipalities to hire medical health officers. The inspection of milk production and distribution facilities was the responsibility of a patchwork of provincial and municipal public health authorities who operated under local dairy inspection regimens. In the 1920s some of these regimes were well funded and developed; others were not.[1]

As outlined in the previous chapter, the 1920s was a time of transition with regard to infant feeding habits, with greater emphasis being put on cow's milk and infant formulas (which were often diluted with cow's milk) and less emphasis on breastfeeding (Myres 1981). The timing of this trend was unfortunate because the quality of the milk supply in many regions of Canada was uneven. This dangerous situation led to the Division of Child Welfare developing and disseminating nutrition education guidelines that were directed specifically at expectant and new mothers (see Chapter 5).

---

[1] The federal government, through the Criminal Code (and the Adulteration Act and Dairy Industry Act), was responsible for prosecuting those who deliberately adulterated milk. However, it could not prosecute farmers or milk distributors who knowingly or unknowingly produced and distributed dirty or diseased milk. This was the responsibility of local public health authorities under municipal public health by-laws and provincial public health legislation.

To understand how these guidelines were developed and why they focused on expectant and new mothers and their children, it is necessary to review the links between persistently high rates of infant mortality, the increasingly popular practice of feeding cow's milk to young infants, and the changing image of milk as, after the First World War, dairy products became an increasingly important commodity within Canadian agriculture.

The first section of this chapter describes the relationship between artificial feeding and infant mortality. The next two sections look at the availability of disease-free cow's milk in Canada as well as at the changing image of milk both among the public and among the public health profession. The last section discusses how the change in the image of milk – from dirty and dangerous liquid to vitamin-rich protective food – was central to the milk marketing strategies that, in conjunction with the federal Department of Agriculture, the dairy industry developed in the 1920s.

Artificial Feeding and Infant Mortality

It was well known that artificial feeding in unsanitary conditions generally meant death for an infant (Baumslag and Michels 1993; Fildes 1986; Stuart-Macadam and Dettwyler 1995). In Britain the scientific link between poverty, increased artificial feeding, and infant mortality was established by the turn of the twentieth century. In a classic study of infant mortality among the poor conducted in London at that time, Newman (1906, 260) concluded that "a mother suckling her infant requires nourishment, and it is lack of nourished mothers among the poor – many of whom are half-starved – that leads to the inability to provide milk for their offspring. This, in its turn, leads to early weaning, which involves artificial feeding, which is one of the most difficult undertakings in the tenement homes of the poor. And so it comes about that the early-weaned infant is so often marked for death in infancy."

The links between artificial feeding and infant mortality were also well known in Canada. The industrial revolution and its concomitant social upheaval in Canada provoked increasing pressure for public health and social reform, resulting in the establishment of milk depots that supplied pasteurized milk and the development of child and maternal hygiene divisions in many municipal public health departments (Allen 1971; Moscovitch and Drover 1987; Valverde 1991). As outlined in Chapter 3, these municipal clinics encouraged women to breastfeed, and many of them also made certified and/or pasteurized cow's milk available to women who were unable or unwilling to breastfeed.

Figure 4.1

Infant mortality rate per 1,000 live births in Canada, 1921-45

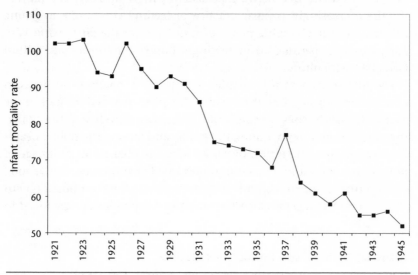

Source: Statistics Canada (1991, Table 2b, 34).

In spite of these efforts, infant mortality rates remained persistently high in Canada throughout the 1920s. For example, in 1921, there were 102.1 infant deaths per 1,000 live births. By 1929 the infant mortality rate was 92.9 per 1,000 live births, a reduction of only 10 percent. However, as Figure 4.1 shows, the decline in infant mortality was uneven over the decade. A clear trend of decreasing infant mortality did not begin in Canada until 1929.

Infant mortality rates were worst among the poor, especially in Canada's large cities and particularly in Montreal (Comacchio 1993). The federal Department of Health was aware that infant mortality rates in Canada were the worst in the industrialized world, noting, in 1921, that the Canadian rate was more than double New Zealand's, which had the lowest rate among developed nations (Canada 1924). There were also huge regional disparities in infant mortality rates across Canada. For example, in 1921 infant mortality ranged from a low of 56.5 per 1,000 live births in British Columbia to a high of 128.0 per 1,000 live births in Quebec (MacMurchy 1923).

Diarrhea constituted one of the main causes of death for children from the mid- to late nineteenth century. In Quebec the common practice of feeding infants broth instead of breast milk was one of the reasons why infant mortality was so high. The broths were often made of a mixture of bread, biscuits, and cornstarch. Apart from providing few nutrients, these broths were likely contaminated by the added water or milk (Bernier 1989). In studies in Montreal conducted near the turn of the twentieth century, it is clear that French Canadian women breastfed much less than did their Irish co-religionists who, in turn, breastfed less than did the city's Anglo-Protestant and Jewish women (Thornton and Olson 1991, 1997, 2001).

In Montreal in the 1890s, each summer poor-quality water and milk caused the deaths of more than 500 infants under one year old. The government attempted to solve these problems by instituting regulations regarding drainage of waste; however, due to lack of inspection and enforcement these regulations were often not followed (Anctil and Bluteau 1986). The much greater infant mortality rates in Quebec were likely due to the extremely low breastfeeding rates among French Canadian women, widespread poverty, and an underdeveloped public health infrastructure.

Availability of Disease-Free Cow's Milk in the 1920s
During the latter quarter of the nineteenth century and the first two decades of the twentieth century rapid industrialization, and the consequent separation of farms from urban consumers, stretched primitive storage and distribution systems. This rendered milk an even greater hazard for poor urban children than it had been for rural children (Cohen and Heimlich 1998). Milk had to be transported long distances and stored for relatively long periods in the absence of refrigeration, and it was often obtained from tuberculosis-infected cattle living on uninspected farms and in unsanitary dairy barns (Dormandy 2000).

This issue was first addressed in Toronto, which, as early as the 1880s, passed laws to regulate dairy barns within the city (MacDougall 1990). It was also addressed relatively early in Quebec City, which adopted regulations on milk distribution and sales in 1893 and, a year later, appointed a milk inspector. In 1899 the authorities suggested inoculating local cows with tuberculin, but it was not until 1907 that this became mandatory. Despite the creation of municipal stables in Quebec City, it remained difficult to control the health of cows and, consequently, the quality of their milk (Anctil 1986).

By 1908 Ottawa had passed stringent by-laws requiring the inspection of all cattle supplying milk to the city, thereby attempting to extend its dairy inspection regimen to rural milk sheds that shipped milk to the city (Hollingsworth 1925). Toronto passed similar laws at this time, and, with growing pressure, in 1911 Ontario passed the Milk Act, which mandated the inspection of herds and dairy facilities province-wide. In 1914, in a further effort to clean the milk supply, Toronto City Council made pasteurization of all milk sold in the city compulsory, so that by the early 1920s milk sold in Toronto was probably safe (MacDougall 1990).

The first province-wide legislation making pasteurization of milk compulsory was not passed until 1938, when Ontario amended its Public Health Act. During the 1920s and 1930s only fifty municipalities of the eight hundred in the province had passed by-laws requiring the pasteurization of all milk offered for sale (MacDougall 1990). As late as 1922 the head of the National Dairy Council of Canada told a meeting of the Canadian Public Health Association that "milk sold in Ontario for domestic consumption (that is, outside of our larger cities), is disgusting, dirty and dangerous" (Stonehouse 1922a, 298). In an article in the *Public Health Journal* he warned that farmers, milk processors, and distributors must continue to be educated and that, in order to maintain current standards and to further improve the cleanliness of milk, there had to be greater cooperation between producers and medical health officers (Stonehouse 1922b).

Five thousand three hundred and fifty-three people were afflicted by Montreal's 1927 typhoid epidemic. The cause of the epidemic was contaminated milk, the result of municipal health officers' being unable to force milk producers to follow hygiene regulations. After the epidemic pressure from physicians finally forced the provincial government to make the pasteurization of milk the responsibility of the provincial Service d'hygiène (Anctil 1986). Nonetheless, in 1929 half of the milk sold in Quebec was still unpasteurized.

Even in Ontario, Canada's most activist public health province, the cleanliness of the milk supply was uneven during the 1920s and 1930s. Outside Ontario, provincial legislation and most municipal by-laws were less advanced. Thus, in spite of better legislation, more inspections of cattle and dairy facilities, and the greater acceptance and availability of pasteurized milk, during the 1920s much of the Canadian milk supply was unclean and potentially dangerous.

Reforming Milk's Image
While most public health professionals had spent the last quarter of the nineteenth century vilifying milk and warning the public of its dangers, by the early 1920s, at least in cities where the milk supply had been cleaned up, these same professionals began to extol the virtues of

milk. Why this about-face? Mainly because of the discovery that vitamins and trace minerals were a necessary part of nutrition, along with fats, proteins, and carbohydrates, and the discovery that milk has a high vitamin and mineral content. These discoveries came quickly between the turn of the century and the early 1920s (Nestle 2002). Foods rich in vitamins were dubbed "protective," and milk was quickly identified as the ideal protective food (Valverde 1991).

As well, in many cases it was from milk that researchers isolated the first vitamins (Rosen 1958). When they broke foods down into protein, fats, and carbohydrates and fed these constituents in pure form to baby animals, these babies died. But when the animals were fed milk, they thrived. Researchers used milk because they knew that, being what young animals ate naturally, it contained all the elements necessary for life.

The publicity around these early vitamin studies was enormous, and the role of milk in these experiments was well publicized. Following the discovery of vitamins, the medical profession was divided over the impact of the pasteurization of cow's milk, some believing that this would denature vitamins, thus negating milk's positive impact on health (Hollingsworth 1925). Once it was discovered that pasteurization only minimally affected vitamin content, public health professionals realized that combined municipal regimens of farm and dairy inspection and pasteurization would make milk safe and, therefore, an ideal protective food.

Thus the early 1920s was a transition time for Canadian milk. On the one hand, because of uneven cleanliness, milk was still dangerous; on the other hand, it was quickly becoming known as the ideal protective food, particularly for children. In order to understand milk's new image it is necessary to consider the economics of the dairy industry, which was also in transition.

New Alliances between the Department of Agriculture, the Dairy Industry, and Public Health Professionals

In 1917, towards the end of the First World War, the federal government passed the War Measures Act, thus creating a centralized Food Control System (Hanna 1917). In an effort to increase the efficiency of milk production and distribution, the food controller formed a milk committee, which recommended consolidating the dairy industry, particularly its milk-distribution component. The committee suggested that having fewer producers and distributors would increase efficiency, ensuring that farmers would obtain better prices and, therefore, have greater incentive to increase production. Fewer producers and distributors would

Figure 4.2

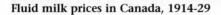

Fluid milk prices in Canada, 1914-29

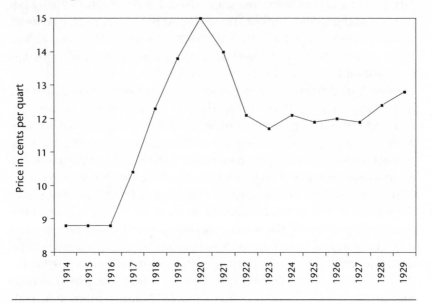

Source: Dominion Bureau of Statistics (1960).

also, of course, make it easier to effectively inspect milk production (Hanna 1917).

While calling for increased consolidation in the milk industry, with the slogan "Patriotism, Production, and Prosperity" the Department of Agriculture also spearheaded a drive to increase wartime agricultural production for export. This resulted in greatly expanded dairy capacity, which peaked just as the war ended and export markets dried up (Britnell and Fowke 1962, 48). The abrupt shift to dependence on the domestic consumption of milk, butter, and cheese at the end of the war occurred during a time of growing food price inflation. This restricted the ability of domestic consumers to purchase dairy products, putting the industry into crisis.[2] As shown in Figure 4.2, the price of milk increased from 8.8 cents per quart in 1914 to a high of 15 cents in 1920. For the duration of the decade it hovered at 12 cents, which was approximately 40 percent higher than it had been at the beginning of the war (Dominion Bureau of Statistics 1960).

[2] Dupuis (2002, 114) has shown that, in the United States, the dairy industry faced similar pressures at the end of the First World War.

Milk consumption was highly sensitive to income. The Food Controller's Milk Committee (Hanna 1917, 6) reported that "any slight increase in the price of milk, unfortunately, has been followed by a largely decreased consumption." Given the inflationary conditions at that time, the committee recommended that "a campaign of education be undertaken, emphasizing the relatively high food value of milk and the many ways of using it. Such a campaign could, perhaps, best be carried out by teachers of Domestic Science and by Home Economics Associations" (ibid.).

This committee and the dairy industry realized that consumption could be increased by reforming the negative image of milk among the public and among public health professionals. But the authors of this report understood that enhancing milk's image would take more than a public relations campaign. They suggested that the dairy industry work more cooperatively with public health professionals to ensure the cleanliness of the milk supply.

Prior to this time, the process of making milk supplies safe had often involved conflict between dairy farmers, processors, and distributors on the one hand, and municipal public health officers on the other, as the latter battled to regulate and to convince the industry of the role dirty milk played in spreading disease (Hollingsworth 1925). The process of educating and cajoling the dairy industry into safer practices involved compromise as well as conflict, both within the industry and between public health and industry officials. As a result, by 1920 in many cities public health professionals and the dairy industry had a long history of working together. As early as 1917 the dairy industry began to campaign hard among its producers, processors, and distributors to improve the cleanliness of the milk supply, associating itself with public health officials, nutritionists, and dieticians to promote the protective benefits of milk to children (*Report of the Milk Committee* 1917).

An early example of this occurred in Toronto in 1922 in an extremely well publicized joint campaign by the Canadian Public Health Association, the Child Welfare Council, and the National Dairy Council of Canada. These groups sponsored Milk Week, specifically targeting schoolchildren and their mothers, in order to promote the increased consumption of milk (Canada 1923). The campaign stressed that milk was rich in vitamins and minerals and that it had special protective effects on children's health. The message was spread by politicians, public health officials, and National Dairy Council officials, all of whom gave speeches, attended carnivals in local parks, and participated in parades.

For public health professionals working in cities with clean milk, this 360-degree change in attitude made good health sense, particularly at this stage, when the potential health problems associated with the high fat content of milk were not yet known. For the dairy industry, given the decreasing milk consumption following the war, the recognition of the vitamin and mineral content of milk, and its promotion as a protective food, provided a golden marketing opportunity. However, as will be seen in the next chapter, for medical and nutritional professionals attempting to generate nationwide nutritional advice regarding the reduction of infant mortality, the conflict over milk's mixed reputation and changing status resulted in the proffering of ambivalent advice.

As well as the direct relationships between municipal public health professionals and the Dairy Industry, in 1923 the Department of Agriculture established alliances with the Division of Child Welfare, national child welfare, and women's organizations that were campaigning to increase the "use of milk for children and mothers" (Canada 1923, 42). In 1926 the department, through its Milk Utilization Branch, instituted a milk consumption promotion policy, which entailed "cooperating with public health nurses and child welfare workers; assisting in provincial schemes such as better farming; addressing dairy conventions meetings of school teachers and also public, collegiate and normal school classes. No opportunity is lost for disseminating information as to the dietary value of milk and its products" (Department of Agriculture 1926, 34).

The Milk Utilization Branch began to produce its own nutrition teaching materials. By 1927 it was engaged in "the work of increasing the consumption of dairy products by arousing public interest in their nutritional value. Recognizing the school as an effective medium, normal schools were visited and the teachers-in-training told of the health teaching material available through the service" (Department of Agriculture 1927, 86). At this time dieticians were "employed in this work, had booths for demonstration purposes at the leading exhibitions, attended meetings of health and child welfare organizations, women's institutes, dairy conventions and other similar gatherings. A phase of the work which seems to be popular as well as effective is in connection with the schools – public schools to reach children, and normal schools to interest and instruct prospective teachers" (ibid., 40). Thus, by the late 1920s the Department of Agriculture had forged strong links with children's and women's health organizations and the Division of Child Welfare, and had developed highly targeted milk promotion campaigns that were delivered by professional nutritionists and dieticians and that used health claims based mainly on the vitamin content of milk.

Summary

In the early 1920s both the dairy industry and officials in the Department of Agriculture began to actively promote the domestic consumption of fluid milk. The new science of nutrition, which enthusiastically espoused milk as the quintessential protective food, was used by these interests, and new alliances were made with public health professionals (the purpose being to garner their support for increased milk consumption among children).

During the 1920s and 1930s the dairy industry and public health officials both cooperated and disagreed over issues regarding the safety of the milk supply. Across Canada the cleanliness of milk was uneven. Infant mortality rates, which had been scientifically linked to the ingestion of unclean milk, remained high throughout the 1920s, and the national milk supply was not yet effectively regulated. It was against the confusing backdrop of the increasing public perception of the safety and health-giving qualities of cow's milk and the questionable safety of the milk supply that officials in the Department of Health's Child Welfare Division made its first foray into nutrition education. This is the subject of Chapter 5.

5

The First National Infant Feeding Guidelines in Canada

With the formation of the Division of Child Welfare in 1920, many advocates and professionals requested information on a range of topics related to child health. The division published a series of "Little Blue Books" for Canadian women in general and for mothers in particular (Dodd 1991).

By far the most popular publication produced by the division was *The Canadian Mother's Book* (*CMB*) (MacMurchy 1923). Over 12,000 copies of the first edition of the *CMB* were distributed in 1921. Published in both French and English, 800,000 copies of the 1921, 1923, 1927, and 1932 editions, all edited and revised by Helen MacMurchy, were produced. This amounted to one copy of the *CMB* for every four births in Canada during this eleven-year period (Lewis and Watson 1991/92).

Registrars of births in all provinces and territories sent postcards to new mothers, encouraging them to mail the cards back to the Department of Health for a free copy of the *CMB*. Every mother who requested a copy received one (Lewis and Watson 1991/92). The *CMB*, in various editions, has remained a standard resource for public health professionals, midwives, nurses, doctors, and the lay public from 1921 to the present.

During the interwar years the Child Welfare Division saw the mother as key to reducing infant mortality: "Concentrate on the mother. We must glorify, dignify, and purify motherhood by every means in our power" (McConnachie 1983, 64). Motherhood was the means through which women were to find fulfillment. If the security of the home and the nation depended on raising healthy children, then motherhood was a national duty.

Breastfeeding and the practice of sound mothering would reduce infant mortality. The first national dietary guidelines issued by the division regarding the feeding of pregnant women, mothers, and infants were published in the *CMB*. The editions from the 1920s preached the centrality of the mother in breastfeeding – a message echoed in La Leche League publications once that organization emerged some forty year later. Throughout the 1920s the tone and content of these booklets reflected the major battles under way between physicians, pediatricians, and nursing and other public health professionals, particularly with regard to breastfeeding and artificial feeding.

The first section of this chapter looks at the dietary advice that the *CMB* offered pregnant women and mothers. The next section discusses the conflicting messages found in the *CMB*s during the 1920s, and the third section addresses the changing infant feeding advice in light of new research on the link between vitamin D and rickets. The final section evaluates the role of the Child Welfare Division in developing breastfeeding education programs during the 1920s.

The Canadian Mother's Book

After the discovery of vitamins, dietary advice was increasingly concerned not just with ensuring adequate energy intake and balanced consumption of carbohydrates, fats, and protein but also with problems of vitamin deficiency. Accordingly, protective foods, rich in essential vitamins, were seen as especially important to ensure health through pregnancy and labour and to ensure the mother's strength through a long period of breastfeeding, thereby reducing infant mortality.

As the experts in the Division of Child Welfare assumed that all mothers could and would breastfeed their infants until nine months of age, advice on artificial feeding was not contained in the early editions of the *CMB*. In fact, advice on artificial feeding did not appear in the *CMB* until 1940. And, in that year, for the first time, the length of time advised for exclusive breastfeeding was reduced from nine months to six months.

The editions of the *CMB* produced in the 1920s recommended a variety of foods for the expectant mother, including cereals, bread and biscuits, vegetables, fruit, meat, fish, eggs, and soup. It advised expectant mothers to roast, boil, or broil meat or fish once a day; to eat butter or cream two or three times daily; to avoid fatty meats and fish or vegetables fried in fat; and to eat fruit, vegetables, and cereals two or three times a day. Advice on avoiding fatty meats and fish or vegetables fried in fat stemmed from the belief, prevalent at the time, that fats "should not be taken in excess in pregnancy as patients may complain of heartburn" (McIlroy 1938, 95). In sum, the *CMB* (MacMurchy 1923, 19) advised expectant mothers to eat and drink "much liquid, plenty of vegetables, salads, fruit, cereals, not too much meat, fish or fat" – advice that is fairly consistent with today's dietary guidelines.

The *CMB* was ambivalent about milk. It issued dire warnings to mothers about feeding cow's milk to babies under nine months of age and strongly advocated breastfeeding, stating that the mother "knows her nursing is the greatest safeguard for the baby's life. She knows that her milk will not only nourish him but protect him from many of the diseases of infancy. She does not want her baby to die. Nursing the baby is the easiest way. No formula with bottles and rubber nipples, and measuring spoons and milk-sugar and sterilizing, and no one knows what else, for the Canadian Mother. These things will get dirty and dirt in milk is death to the baby" (MacMurchy 1923, 72).

The *CMB* (MacMurchy 1923, 82) advised mothers to drink cow's milk only after their babies were born and to "keep on the same diet that suited you before the baby came but drink a great deal more – say a pint or more of milk a day and plenty of water three or four times a day. You should have meat at one meal every day. Milk is our greatest protective food. You must have it."

After clearly warning Canadian mothers away from feeding milk to babies under nine months of age, the *CMB* (MacMurchy 1923, 107) described the role of milk in the diet of babies older than nine months as follows: "Milk is the indispensable food for children. They cannot do without it. The cow has been well called the 'the foster mother of the human race.' Little children must have milk to enable them to grow properly. No matter what it costs, milk is still the cheapest food for children. Children from nine months to two years should have about two pints of milk every day in addition to other food, and it is really a mistake to give them any less till they are about twelve years of age. Three large cups of milk a day is the very least they should have."

The *CMB* repeatedly counselled that milk for babies over nine months of age should be pasteurized, stored properly, and dirt-free, reflecting the extreme unease that professionals in the Division of Child Welfare felt about the safety of the milk supply. As the next section shows, the public health, pediatric, and child welfare specialists in the Division of Child Welfare did not trust physicians and nurses to dispense sound dietary advice to Canadian mothers.

Role of the Physicians and Nurses in Breastfeeding and Artificial Feeding

The first editions of the *CMB* clearly laid out the roles of mother, father, nurse, and doctor in the breastfeeding process. Placing the mother and support for the mother at the centre, the *CMB* (MacMurchy 1923, 70) states: "It is to the Canadian Mother that we look for leadership in Child Welfare and especially in establishing Maternal Nursing as the Canadian Way." While the mother was seen as the leader, "the Father, the Doctor, the Nurse, the rest of the family and all us Canadians must help the Mother to make Maternal Nursing the Canadian Way" (74).

In the second edition of the *CMB* (MacMurchy 1923, 74), women were warned that, "since the first edition of the *Canadian Mother's Book* was published, we have received information showing that, in too many cases, Doctors and Nurses are responsible for the baby being taken from the Mother's breast and fed artificially." According to the *CMB*, the "doctor depends on the Nurse to manage the nursing" and the "doctor is responsible for seeing that the Nurse manages it [the nursing] properly and advises the Mother wisely" (ibid.).

The *CMB* aggressively promoted breastfeeding by raising the spectre of infant death arising from artificial feeding and, in particular, from the use of cow's milk and infant formulas. At the same time it exhorted mothers to be wary of the medical profession. Mothers were warned that some physicians (and, to a lesser extent, nurses) were unreliable breastfeeding advocates. According to the *CMB* physicians should have an arm's-length role in the breastfeeding process. They were to instruct the nurses, who should be the ones directly advising and guiding breastfeeding mothers. The nurses were to manage the mothers, but in a respectful and supportive way, so that the mothers would remain in control of the breastfeeding process.

The Division of Child Welfare's breastfeeding guidelines were comprehensive and included information for mothers on how to engage with medical professionals in order to support the process. These guidelines were fairly consistent in the various editions of the *CMB* published during the interwar years. However, after 1940 the breastfeeding focus of the *CMB*s was steadily eroded until the 1970s, when, with the women's movement and the growth in popularity of pronatal organizations such as the La Leche League, breastfeeding guidelines made a 180-degree turn back to mother-supported breastfeeding (Myres 1979, 1981).

The way in which infants were fed was not only important with regard to preventing infant mortality but was also closely linked to many of the nutritional deficiency diseases of infancy, particularly rickets.

Rickets and *The Canadian Mother's Book*
Rickets was a disease recognized over 300 years ago in Britain. By the eighteenth century folk healers and some doctors realized that it could

be both prevented and cured by exposing a child to sunlight and/or administering cod-liver oil (Goldbloom 1945).[1] While people did not know what substances in cod-liver and other fish oils prevented and cured rickets, these substances were often administered to children. Rickets was almost always associated with poverty and malnutrition and was usually found in children under two years of age. And it was more common among artificially fed infants than it was among those who had been breastfed.

In Canada until the 1930s, when it began to decline, rickets was a devastating disease that killed hundreds of children each year and left thousands with life-long deformities. It is difficult to know how widespread rickets was in Canada before 1926, when mortality statistics became available in all provinces. Between 1926 and 1929 the disease caused approximately 200 deaths per year (see Chapter 7) (Dominion Bureau of Statistics, 1921-50).

In 1920 the British Medical Research Council was formed, and its first research project involved a study of childhood rickets conducted by Edward Mellanby. Prior to the First World War Mellanby had discovered that a fat-soluble vitamin in butter and cod-liver oil, later isolated as Vitamin D, prevented and cured rickets in animals. Conclusive scientific proof was provided in 1923, when researchers in Vienna demonstrated that supplemental feeding of cod-liver oil or exposing the skin to strong sunshine could cure severe rickets in children.

When the first few editions of the *CMB* were published, the role of vitamins was not well understood. Although vitamins were known to be important, their role in the etiology of rickets and scurvy was unclear. Nonetheless, these early editions did advise mothers to supplement breast milk with fruit juice – either strained orange, apple, or prune juice – when the infant was one month old for "health reasons" and in order to prevent constipation. This advice was negated to some extent in the early editions, at least in relation to the prevention of rickets, as they also advised mothers to keep their children away from sunlight.

Mellanby's research was disseminated rapidly, and by the late 1920s Canadian health authorities knew that "rickets is a disease of Nutrition caused by lack of Sun and lack of Suitable Food. Rickets may be easily prevented by Sun, Suitable Food and Cod Liver Oil" (MacMurchy 1929, 3).

---

[1] No less an authority than Sir William Osler was aware of this treatment in nineteenth-century Canada as he recommended that, daily, children be taken outside and have their diets supplemented with cod-liver oil (Wilton 1995).

In 1926 the Division of Child Welfare incorporated this new research into its guidelines. That year the *CMB* recommended that mothers administer two or three drops of cod-liver oil twice a day, beginning at one week of age. This dosage was to be gradually increased to two teaspoonfuls twice a day from the age of four to twenty-four months between October first and May first (MacMurchy 1929).

By 1928 the Division of Child Welfare began to advise mothers to give their children regular sunbaths, stipulating that "as the weather gets warmer the Baby may stay out longer. Slight tanning is a good sign" (MacMurchy 1929, 15). This advice reversed earlier proscriptions that mothers "keep the baby out in the air as much as possible, but not in the sun" (MacMurchy 1923, 88). By the late 1920s the *CMB* was still advising women to exclusively breastfeed for nine months, but it suggested supplementing this regimen with cod-liver oil, fruit juice, and sunbaths.

Role of the Division of Child Welfare in Disseminating Nutrition Advice in the 1920s

The *CMB*'s advice was, by and large, the product of the reform movements that had come about due to frustration with the negative impacts of industrialization, especially on the urban poor. These movements, broadly inspired by the social gospel movement and women's fight for the vote, produced an ideology that focused on mother-centred breastfeeding. This ideology was both essentialist and feminist, and its patriotic tone linked breastfeeding with woman's "natural" role as a mother – a role that was linked to nation building.

This major national effort to promote breastfeeding began just as women were beginning to abandon it in droves. According to Myres (1981, 1078), Canadian physicians were only partly responsible for the move away from breastfeeding: "governments, health care professionals, hospitals, the infant formula industry and women themselves have all at one time or another been held responsible for the decline in breastfeeding in the twentieth century." The decline in breastfeeding from the 1920s to the late 1960s was a phenomenon that was observed in many nations other than Canada, and it had complex roots, one of which was the active involvement of many medical professionals in promoting artificial feeding. Also, many women, particularly educated women, wanted alternatives to breastfeeding and enthusiastically embraced artificial infant feeding because it was linked with progressive, scientific, and modern thinking about child rearing. While the steadfast defence of breastfeeding offered through the *CMBs* was undoubtedly the best advice from a health point of view, it was also likely ineffective in stemming the move away from breastfeeding during the interwar years.

It is not clear how practical the *CMBs* advice was for poor working women. The national campaign to promote breastfeeding gave little guidance to those women who needed to work and for whom breastfeeding was not a viable alternative. These women often fed their children artificially in less than hygienic conditions, and what they needed was clean cow's milk and clean water. Nonetheless, while largely ignored, the breastfeeding advice promulgated by national authorities throughout the 1920s and 1930s served to remind health professionals and the public about the importance of breastfeeding.

While exclusive breastfeeding for infants under nine months of age may have been the best advice, the standard setters in the Child Welfare Division lent their support to the aggressive milk promotion campaigns that were undertaken in conjunction with the dairy industry and the Department of Agriculture (see Chapter 4). This gave the public a double message and undermined the breastfeeding standard.

The Child Welfare Division promoted the use of cow's milk among schoolchildren and, thus, effectively lent its support to the improvement of milk's image and to marketing it through health and vitamin claims. This likely also contributed to making cow's milk more acceptable for infants under nine months. The *CMB*'s stance that, on the one hand, cow's milk was highly unsafe for infants under the age of nine months while, on the other hand, it was perfectly safe for those over the age of nine months, reflected the confusion and the uneasy compromise between the Child Welfare Division and its partners in the Department of Agriculture and the dairy industry.

While the breastfeeding advice in the *CMBs* of the late 1920s was sound, it was largely ignored. The increasing availability of clean milk, the increased contact between the medical profession and expectant and new mothers, the growing popularity of artificial formulas, and women's desire to embrace modernity by moving away from traditional breastfeeding habits all contributed to a significant change in infant feeding practices – a change that accelerated in the 1930s.

Summary

In the early 1920s the first dietary guidelines were developed by the Division of Child Welfare in order to improve the nutrition of pregnant women and their infants and, most important, to encourage breastfeeding and thus reduce infant mortality. The division was established following forty years of activism on the part of women's groups, church groups, and trade unionists, who worked together to reduce poverty, to improve working conditions, to effect social and urban reform, and to bring about women's suffrage. The dietary guidelines placed mothers at the centre of the breastfeeding process and kept medical professionals at arm's length.

Throughout the 1920s the dietary guidelines emphatically promoted breastfeeding for at least the first nine months of a baby's life and warned mothers away from cow's milk or infant formulas. Still, they reflected a certain ambivalence about cow's milk, touting it as an ideal protective food for children over nine months of age but as dangerous to those under that age. In the early 1920s the Child Welfare Division moved very quickly to develop joint milk promotion campaigns with the Department of Agriculture. These campaigns were aimed at increasing the consumption of milk, particularly among children, and they used messages produced by nutritional professionals to reinforce the idea that milk was the most important protective food.

In 1926 the division began advising mothers to regularly administer cod-liver oil (and regular sun baths) to breastfeeding infants in order to prevent rickets. By the beginning of the Depression, nutrition guidelines for expectant and new mothers and their babies and young children had been widely disseminated in Canada, in both English and French.

Breastfeeding guidelines were issued at a time of scientific excitement over the newly discovered value of milk and its role in protecting against undernutrition and promoting optimal health. The public's enthusiasm for the new science of nutrition, patchwork improvements in the safety of cow's milk, and the dairy industry's and Department of Agriculture's promotion of the protective benefits of milk compromised the ability of the Division of Child Welfare to deliver the best possible dietary guidelines.

With the Depression, prices for most agricultural commodities fell drastically. As the Depression deepened, these early efforts at nutrition policy became ever more closely tied to the needs of an agricultural industry in crisis. This is outlined in the next chapter, as are changes in the food safety system and in the role of the medical profession with regard to dispensing nutritional advice during the 1930s.

6

Food Safety and Marketing and the Role of the Medical Profession in Dispensing Nutritional Advice in the 1930s

The Division of Child Welfare was shut down, due to budget cuts, in 1933. In 1938 it was resurrected as the Division of Child and Maternal Hygiene. In the intervening years, some of the division's work was temporarily transferred to small, underfunded non-governmental organizations such as the Canadian Council on Child and Maternal Welfare (Burns 1967). Accordingly, during the worst years of the Depression, information about food and nutrition came mainly from the Department of Agriculture. As the Depression deepened, the department increased its research and developed more graded meat and dairy products, aiming both to increase the quality of food and to more efficiently market it to consumers with high disposable income. During the 1930s, as the decline in infant mortality rates accelerated, the focus of the medical profession shifted from infants to their mothers. This was due to persistently high maternal mortality rates, which remained unchanged in Canada until the invention of sulphonamide antibiotics in 1937 (Couture 1939, 1940).

During the Depression the strains on the national food safety, inspection, and surveillance system increased. The vitamin mania of the 1920s laid the foundation for misadvertising campaigns based on health claims. As the Depression deepened, and as competition in the food business grew more intense, old methods of adulteration were resurrected and new ones invented. This occurred against the backdrop of an agricultural economy that moved increasingly from plant- to animal-based production and a need to market relatively expensive animal-based foods to the population. Economic hardship in the agricultural sector was particularly severe, and it shaped the scope and character of the intense food-marketing campaigns undertaken during this time.

The first section in this chapter discusses the economic impact of the Depression. The second section describes the evolution of the food safety system in the 1920s and the 1930s, while the third section outlines the impact of the Depression on agriculture and shows how this shaped domestic food marketing strategies. The final section outlines the impact of changing patterns of physician and hospital utilization, and shows how these consolidated the medical profession's role as the key dispensers of infant feeding advice.

Economic Impact of the Depression

The Wall Street crash in October 1929 triggered an international economic depression, which, in Canada, reached its nadir in 1933, flattening the agricultural sector. The impact of the Depression was disproportionately borne by the agricultural sector and exacerbated the already structurally weak position of Canadian farmers. Between 1929 and 1933 agriculture's share of national income fell from 23 percent to 12 percent, while the proportions earned from the manufacturing and service sectors remained stable (Friesen 1987, 385). Paradoxically, the drastic decline in prices for agricultural produce that occurred in 1929 (because exports were throttled and because domestic incomes plummeted) did not stifle agricultural output (Drummond et al. 1966). According to the Agricultural Economics Research Council of Canada, "this seemingly perverse response of supply to a decline in demand resulted from a lack of non-farm employment opportunities, which served to increase the number of self-employed persons in agriculture; thus farm production was maintained and in some cases actually increased" (ibid., 33).

In 1934 the economy began to revive, and by 1939 it had recovered to levels typical of the late 1920s. As well, although the economic impacts of the Depression were severe, they were unevenly distributed. While conditions were hard for the unemployed, those who remained employed "suffered no reduction in real income. Most of the workers in the skilled trades, the professions and the white-collar occupations who retained their jobs actually enjoyed a considerable improvement in their real position" (Horn 1972, 168). Further, the price of food and other goods plummeted so that, paradoxically, by 1939 the relative cost of living for many Canadians was very low.

In response to deep, prolonged, and historically unprecedented structural unemployment, all levels of government (as well as private charities) initiated relief efforts, especially in western Canada. In the Prairie provinces "churches, welfare organizations in the rest of Canada distributed thousands of rail car loads of fruit, vegetables, clothing, fuel, and blankets during the decade" (Friesen 1987, 394). As well, in the Prairie provinces and British Columbia labour camps were established to provide work and food and to control the growing army of young, single, unemployed males.

While the federal government did not establish a permanent unemployment relief system until the 1940s (see Chapter 9), it intervened reluctantly, slowly, and in piecemeal fashion during the 1930s with temporary loans and grants to bolster the finances of municipal and provincial governments, which were faltering under the burden of providing long-term relief for unemployed workers. As the Depression deepened, the work of the food safety, inspection, and surveillance system was transformed. These changes had begun earlier in the 1920s, with the growing popularity of vitamins and the consequent growth in opportunities to use false health claims to sell food.

New Pressures on the Food Safety System

The work of the food inspectorate was directed mainly towards controlling the imports of butter, fruit, spices, meat, and nuts. These products accounted for approximately 40 percent of the samples tested during the 1920s. Spices, fruit, and nuts were almost all imported from abroad, and most of the butter inspections appear to have been directed against imports of Australian, New Zealand, American, and Fijian butter (Department of Health 1921-25; Department of Pensions and National Health, 1926-30).

While the inspectorate was export- and import-focused, criminal prosecutions brought by the Food and Drug Division were largely for domestic infractions. Throughout the 1920s the average yearly number of prosecutions was 125 (Department of Health and Department of Pensions and National Health Reports 1921-29). Approximately one-third of these were launched to discourage the adulteration of meat. The most common problem involved the addition of sulphite to meat (mainly sausage) to improve its colour and to slow decomposition. Most prosecutions were directed at domestic meat producers. During this decade one-third of all prosecutions resulted in a conviction, but departmental reports contain no information on the identities of those prosecuted or convicted (i.e., it is not clear whether the target of inspectors was retailers, wholesalers, or manufacturers).

Laboratory work also increased during the 1920s, with a fourfold increase in the number of samples processed. To cope with this increase in volume new branch laboratories were opened in Montreal in 1923 and in Toronto in 1927. The rise of mass food marketing through chain stores and the increasing presence of canned and packaged foods in stores meant that the laboratories were conducting more and more bacteriological analyses. In order to handle the sophisticated bacteriological examinations required for canned and packaged food, the Food and Drug Division established a new laboratory in 1925.

In 1927 the Food and Drug Act was amended and consolidated, with heavy borrowing from similar British and American acts and with input from Canadian manufacturers. Amendments included regulations for food labels on all packages weighing more than two ounces (an increasingly important issue, what with the proliferation of canned and packaged goods). Following this amendment, the Food and Drug Division's responsibilities began to shift, with "greater emphasis laid on advertising and labelling with the result that instances of misbranding far outstripped those of adulteration" (Davidson 1949, 78).

The arrival of the Depression in 1929 increased pressure on the agency as the economic crisis, in combination with new technological and food marketing challenges, resulted in adulteration infractions becoming "more numerous in times such as those through which we have been passing. Business competition has been exceptionally keen, with the inevitable result of the tendency to cheapen products without regard to quality. Old forms of food adulteration have been revived and numerous devices of a surprising character have been initiated" (Department of Pensions and National Health 1933, 44).

While misbranding basically involved the inaccurate or fraudulent description of what was contained in cans or packages of food, it also often involved unsubstantiated or false health claims. False claims for vitamins – particularly for vitamins added to breakfast cereals – emerged as a major issue in 1929 as manufacturers began to add vitamins to their products and to make unrealistic health claims for them: "The day had dawned when the commercial potentialities of those substances [vitamins] were being recognized. The unbridled nature of the claims made some control necessary in the public interest" (Davidson 1949, 76).

Accordingly, in 1934, in response to an alarming increase in health claims involving vitamins, an amendment to the Food and Drug Act was passed. Although the Food and Drug Division had been screening newspaper advertisements for false claims relating to food labels since the late 1920s, with the establishment of the CBC in 1933 it also began screening food advertisements broadcast on the radio. The Food and Drug Division also established a vitamin analysis unit: "The scope of the new laboratory, established in 1937, was to investigate claims for vitamin products and examine their potencies" (Davidson 1949, 77).

And, "on account of increasing manufacture and sale by commercial houses of foods and drugs containing vitamins, it is urgently required that their control be closely supervised to prevent exploitation of the public. Such control has required an extension to the present laboratory quarters and an increase in the number of technical assistants" (Department of Pensions and National Health 1937, 19).

Increased sharpness of competition, under Depression-era conditions, drove retailers and manufacturers to develop new forms of fraud. Expanding on the time-honoured practice of adding filler or illegal preservatives to a product in an attempt to directly cheat their customers, the new technologies of canning and retailing made the label a powerful weapon that, in the absence of regulatory controls, was increasingly being used to sell products on the basis of false content and/or health claims. These attempts at fraud necessitated the expansion of laboratory facilities and a shift towards the inspection of food labels and advertisements.

During the 1930s, while the Food and Drug Division was overseeing an increasingly sophisticated and comprehensive food surveillance system, another branch of the Department of Health, the Division of Child Welfare, took a back seat in nutrition education as the severe economic conditions put the Department of Agriculture in the driver's seat.

Marketing Milk and Meat during the Depression

After 1930, when the American government passed the Smoot-Hawley tariff banning imports of agricultural products from Canada, the Department of Agriculture intensified its efforts to develop the domestic market for Canadian foodstuffs. Historically low prices for grain during the 1930s led to increased animal production, which exacerbated surpluses for dairy products and meat, placing downward pressure on prices. In response, the department increased the pace of milk and meat promotion (Britnell and Fowkes 1962).

The Department of Agriculture produced publications with titles such as "Healthful Meals at Low Cost," which emphasized "the importance of including in low-cost meals, sufficient milk, butter and cheese to protect health and promote growth" (Department of Agriculture 1933, 31). Milk promotion intensified even further as, in 1938, the department developed milk foundations across Canada, which were patterned after similar organizations in the United States. These foundations were established to "bring the producers and distributors of fluid milk together in a joint sponsorship of a health and nutrition education program"

(Department of Agriculture 1933). In this way, marketing boards, newly formed in some provinces due to farmer militancy (which arose from price squeezes), were brought into the health-based milk promotion campaigns.

At the same time, the Department of Agriculture increased its research and quality control and, especially for dairy products and beef, began intensively promoting the sale of graded products. The process of dividing milks, cheeses, butters, and various meats into different grades improved quality control, which likely increased the quality and safety of these foods. Grading also provided opportunities for micro-marketing as better-quality products could be priced higher and sold to those with more disposable income.

The department's grading strategy increasingly involved beef, particularly after 1935, when prices dropped to their lowest levels in the twentieth century (see Chapter 7). As early as 1930 "considerable progress ha[d] been made in informing Canadian consumers regarding the nature and value of the Beef Grading Service" (Department of Agriculture 1931, 63). And, in the middle of the Depression, "the consumer appreciates the advantage of being able to purchase beef which carries official identification of quality and is attested by the fact that sales of graded beef during the year 1933 were approximately 50 per cent higher than for the year 1932, and also double sales of 1931. The steadily increasing demand for graded beef suggests the possibilities in developing the domestic market as an incentive to the production and finishing of the best class of beef cattle" (Department of Agriculture 1934, 41).

By the late 1930s, as the Depression began to ease, the Department of Agriculture was reorganized and "a broader program covering all Canadian agricultural food products was undertaken with a view to giving consumers information regarding the nutritive value of various Canadian food products and the facts about graded food products" (Department of Agriculture 1939).

With the elimination of the Division of Child Welfare in the latter part of the 1930s, the Department of Agriculture took the lead in nutrition education, motivated by the need to promote sales of dairy products and meat as livestock, particularly dairy herds, expanded rapidly following the First World War. While the department effectively used current science (particularly the new science of vitamins) in many of its marketing campaigns, the medical profession, also using arguments based on science and technological progress, began to take a larger role in nutrition education.

The Medical Profession and Nutrition Education in the 1930s

The advent of automobiles and the building of highways in the 1920s and 1930s increased access to general practitioners. This was important because, at this time, approximately half of Canadians lived in rural areas. However, the life of a general practitioner in rural Canada was not easy as medical fees remained flat from the 1890s until the 1920s, despite a threefold increase in the wholesale price index (Urquhart and Buckley 1965). Collecting fees from patients was particularly difficult in rural areas because many of the patients were poor, and bills often remained uncollected.

The Depression exacerbated this situation. During the 1930s, in some regions of Ontario fee collection rates fell to an average of 35 percent (Shortt 1981). In harder hit regions of the country, like Saskatchewan, physicians often bartered their services for food (MacLeod and MacLeod 1987). Physicians' incomes plummeted and did not return to 1920s levels until the middle of the Second World War. Physicians across Canada were in dire economic straights, and competition for paying patients intensified.

During the interwar years women of means who were of child-bearing age were increasingly encouraged to use hospitals to give birth, usually on the private wards. Due to concern about seemingly intractable maternal mortality rates, hospitals began admitting more maternity cases in the 1920s. Many women were persuaded that hospitals were safer places to give birth than was the home, although in the pre-antibiotic era this was a somewhat dubious claim. For example, a major study in Ontario in 1933 demonstrated that maternal mortality rates in the province's hospitals were twice that of home births; and, among rural women, who seldom birthed in hospitals at this time, maternal mortality was much lower than it was for urban women (Ontario Department of Health 1934; Oppenheimer 1983). In 1926, 17.8 percent of births in Canada occurred in hospitals, but by 1940 this had increased to 45.3 percent (Statistics Canada 1983). Vancouver led the way with 92 percent of births in hospitals by 1940 (Gagan and Gagan, 2002).[1] While infant mortality

---

[1] The Second World War further accelerated the shift of birthing from home to hospital. By 1945, 63.2 percent of women gave birth in hospital (Statistics Canada 1983). By 1959, 93.1 percent of all births in Canada occurred in a hospital. Also, in 1954 the birth rate peaked (at 28.5 births per 1,000 women). The combined acceleration in the birth rate and the rate at which birthing shifted to hospitals meant that, by the mid-1950s, approximately 20 percent of all hospital admissions in Canada were maternity cases.

began a long-term decline in Canada, beginning in 1930, maternal mortality remained persistently high (Statistics Canada 1983).

During the 1920s and early 1930s most Canadian experts felt that the key to reducing maternal mortality lay in increased medical supervision of mothers during pregnancy and after birth, with particular emphasis on improved postnatal care and better training in obstetrics (Comacchio 1993; Couture 1939, 1940; Department of Pensions and National Health 1942; Kerr 1935). These ideas were echoed in the various reports on maternal mortality published in Britain and the United States during this time (Titmuss 1938; Williams 1997).

Birthing women's access to hospitals and physicians increased during the 1930s, enhancing the role of physicians and nurses in postnatal care and giving them more influence over infant feeding. This shift occurred against a backdrop of increased conflict between pediatricians and other physicians on the one hand, and nurses and advocates of exclusive breastfeeding on the other.

As physicians gained greater contact with women during their post-natal care in the 1930s, pediatricians in Canada took an international lead in developing better artificial infant foods. Three doctors at the Hospital for Sick Children in Toronto were responsible for inventing several products that promised increased nutritional value for children. One of the first products developed by Allan Brown, Frederick Tisdall, and Theodore Drake was Sunwheat Biscuits, which consisted of whole wheat, wheat germ, milk, butter, yeast, bone meal, iron, and copper. This biscuit was used as a nutritional supplement for toddlers and young children. The McCormick's food company marketed the product in the early 1930s, with all royalties from the sale returning to the hospital for further pediatric research.

Pablum was invented at the Toronto Hospital for Sick Children in 1931. This was the first pre-cooked, vitamin- and mineral-enriched cereal for infants. Consisting of a mixture of wheatmeal, cornmeal, wheat germ, brewer's yeast, bone meal, and alfalfa, it contained five of the six known vitamins (A, B1, B2, D, and E). In 1934 E. Mead Johnson began to market Pablum, with the royalties from its sale returning to the hospital for the next twenty-five years.

Conflict within Medical Practice in Relation to Infant Feeding in the 1930s

The strong language in *The Canadian Mother's Book,* particularly the explicit warnings to mothers to be wary of physicians or nurses who might attempt to undermine their breastfeeding practices, reflected a much broader battle that was taking place between physicians and nurses. By the 1920s the secular nursing profession in Canada, after having been in existence for approximately forty years, had begun to organize itself and to push for more autonomy in relation to hospital administrators and physicians (Ostry 2006).

In the sphere of infant feeding, mother-centred breastfeeding, as outlined in the *CMB*, was approved by most physicians (as long as the physician remained the central authority). However, in the late 1920s nurses began to demand a greater role in the care of patients, including dispensing advice about infant feeding. This erupted into controversy around the establishment of a mothercraft centre in Toronto.

The aim of this centre, which was established in 1931 and was based on a New Zealand nursing model, was to ensure adequate nutrition for infants whose mothers were experiencing challenges initiating or maintaining breastfeeding. The new Toronto centre attempted to counter the "under-nourishment of infants whose mothers [were] desirous of giving them natural feeding, but because of easily correctable reasons [were] unable to do so" (Department of Health 1932). However, the centre raised questions regarding professional authority in the realm of infant feeding. Only physicians had the right to prescribe infant formulas. However, the Mothercraft Centre challenged this. Nurses at the centre were trained in methods developed by Dr. Truby King, an internationally renowned leader in child and maternal welfare. Mothercraft nurses followed the King method completely, including prescribing infant feedings in cases when all attempts at breastfeeding had failed. Physicians were strongly opposed to nurses directly prescribing infant food because this infringed on their authority.

Alan Brown was one of the foremost opponents of the Mothercraft Centre. Although the mothercraft system was not substantially different from his own, he considered it to be inferior. Brown, as the chief advisor to Toronto's Division of Maternal and Child Hygiene, refused to cooperate with the centre. As a result, the University of Toronto's Department of Pediatrics, the Academy of Medicine, and the Hospital for Sick Children also denounced the organization. Throughout the 1930s the balance of responsibilities between physician and nurse continued to be negotiated within this tense environment. Not surprisingly, it was the physicians who prevailed (Commachio 1993).

The increasing involvement in perinatal care, promoted within the context of persistently high maternal mortality, gave physicians, hospitals, and (to a lesser extent) nurses a larger role in dispensing nutritional advice to expectant and new mothers and their babies. This was a change from the 1920s, when midwives and the *CMB* were the main source of nutritional advice for women and when the role of both physicians and hospitals was limited.

Summary

The Depression exacerbated the already weak position of agriculture in Canada's national economy, particularly in the Prairie provinces. In spite of rapid declines in the price of food, domestic agricultural production continued apace and, with the closure of international markets, resulted in food surpluses. Concerns about the possibility of widespread hunger mounted with the unemployment rate. With an urgent need to market animal-based foods, officials in the Department of Agriculture embarked on aggressive promotion campaigns to increase the domestic consumption of milk and meat, specifically targeting housewives and schoolchildren.

The economic hardships of the Depression years, which included closed international agricultural markets and continuing high levels of domestic livestock production, led to an intensification of the Department of Agriculture's marketing campaigns. New grading strategies were developed, which both improved the quality of the food supply and led to better marketing. As well, as the Depression deepened in the mid-1930s, strategies were developed to market to those with lower incomes.

The Depression led to the demise of the Division of Child Welfare in 1933, and for most of the 1930s the Department of Agriculture took the lead in nutrition education. It continued to promote the consumption of meat and dairy products much as it had in the 1920s – through extolling the health benefits of these protective foods.

Meanwhile, the Food and Drug Division faced many new challenges in the late 1920s and 1930s, with the growth of a mass food market for packaged and canned goods, increased advertising, greater consolidation in food retailing, and growing public fascination with (and corporate willingness to exploit) the use of vitamins. As the frequency of food adulteration was increasing during the Depression, the Food and Drug Division shifted its regulatory efforts to the even more rapidly increasing problems of the misbranding of food labels and the touting of false health claims, particularly for products with added vitamins.

In the 1930s, propelled mainly by growing concerns about maternal mortality and the growing difficulty of making a good living, the medical profession obtained greater influence over maternity care and, therefore, a larger role in dispensing nutrition advice to mothers and their infants. Conflict over the role of physicians and nurses in the feeding of infants increased as nurses attempted to take on a stronger role in artificial infant feeding. Also during this time pediatricians in Toronto became international leaders in the development of artificial foods.

As the Depression deepened, fears about ill-health surfaced, particularly among the children of the unemployed. Even though millions suffered in the Depression, paradoxically, the health status of the population improved and the food supply stabilized for some items and increased for others. It is this paradoxical situation to which the next two chapters are devoted.

7

Food Supply during the Depression

During the 1930s the Canadian system of food safety was strengthened, domestic food marketing on the part of industry and agriculture and medical involvement in infant feeding increased, and breastfeeding rates declined. In the ten years between the 1929 stock market crash and the beginning of the Second World War in 1939, the economy contracted, leading to widespread unemployment and economic hardship.

As unemployment deepened calls for a national unemployment program grew, as did pressure on cash-strapped municipal and provincial governments to provide more generous unemployment relief payments. The debate over the amounts paid by local and provincial governments for unemployment relief was increasingly centred on the availability and cost of food, which was the single largest expense for unemployed families (Canadian Preparatory Committee 1936).[1] Concerns about hunger, particularly among the long-term unemployed, and its possible impact on the health of children were also increasingly voiced by reformers and medical experts.

In spite of these mounting concerns, somewhat paradoxically, between 1929 and 1939, the health status of Canadians improved dramatically. In 1931 in Canada the average age at death was 43.1 years. By 1941 it was 51.4 years – an increase of 19.2 percent (Wadhera and Strachan 1993, 238).

The Depression-era improvements in lifespan occurred as death rates from typical diseases of affluence (coronary heart disease and cancer)

---

[1] Dietary surveys undertaken in 1939 showed that middle- and low-income urban Canadians spent from 30 percent to 60 percent of family income on food (Hunter and Pett 1941; Patterson and McHenry 1941; Sylvestre and Nadeau 1941; Young 1941). In the mid-1930s the proportion of family income spent by those on unemployment relief ranged from 60 percent to 80 percent (Grauer 1939).

Figure 7.1

Average death rates per 100,000 population for leading causes of death in Canada, five-year periods, 1921-45

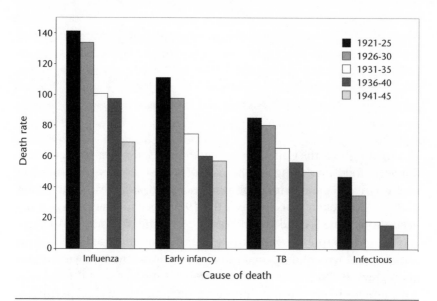

Influenza = influenza, bronchitis, and pneumonia
Early infancy = diseases of early infancy; pneumonia of the newborn is included in both
    "diseases of early infancy" and "influenza, bronchitis and pneumonia" for all years (except
    for the province of Quebec, 1921-25)
TB = tuberculosis
Infectious diseases = diphtheria, whooping cough, measles, scarlet fever, and typhoid fever.
Source: Statistics Canada (1983).

increased rapidly from 1921 to 1940 (Statistics Canada 1983). Increases in these diseases occurred because people were living longer, and they were balanced by major decreases, particularly during the Depression years, in infectious diseases. Figure 7.1 demonstrates sustained declines in infectious disease, particularly in the five-year period when the Depression was at its worst, from 1930 to 1935.

Why did the health of citizens in general, and infants in particular, improve so dramatically during this long decade of economic hardship? Large declines in infant mortality during the 1930s are particularly hard to account for, given the increasing popularity of artificial infant feeding within the context of growing economic insecurity and the associated potential for increased exposure to unsanitary conditions.

The Paradox of Improving Health Status in the 1930s

In discussing infant health improvements in the United States during the first half of the twentieth century, Rima Apple (1987, 172) comments: "it is likely that the rising standard of living, greater access to medical care, and improved food and water supplies ... at least in part masked the negative effects of the growing utilization of artificial infant feeding." This was not likely true either for the United States or for Canada, particularly during the 1930s. In Canada, given that, before the widespread availability of antibiotics in the 1940s, physicians tended to support artificial infant feeding and that clean milk was not evenly available, it is not clear how greater access to physicians (which occurred in the 1930s) would have "masked" the negative effects of artificial feeding.

Apple attributes health improvements in the United States to "rising living standards in the first half of the twentieth century." In Canada, for most of the first half of the twentieth century the economy did not perform well, expanding only between 1900 and 1913, 1926 and 1929, and after 1940. The economy was stagnant through most of the 1920s and contracted during most of the 1930s (Bliss 1987). Improved access to physicians and rising standards of living do not explain improvements in the health status of Canadians during the 1930s.

In an argument pre-dating and somewhat similar to Apple's, Thomas McKeown suggests that rising standards of living were primarily responsible for mortality declines in the British population in the late nineteenth century. He postulates that, as living standards improved, so did the dietary and the nutritional status of the population, thus enhancing resistance to infectious diseases and lowering mortality rates. He also shows that steep declines in mortality from tuberculosis (the main killer in the nineteenth century) were well under way in the decades prior to the availability of effective medical treatment for the disease. Unlike Apple, he concludes that medical care was irrelevant and that the decline in tuberculosis mortality was mainly due to nutritional improvements that enhanced resistance to the disease (McKeown and Brown 1955; McKeown 1976).

McKeown's critics have quite rightly pointed out that the standard of living did not improve in steady fashion in Britain throughout the nineteenth century, partially undermining his basic assumption that improved economic activity led to better diets, which, in turn, led to the decline in tuberculosis mortality. His critics also argue that McKeown's definition of medical care is too narrow as it is based solely on curative care delivered by physicians, thereby excluding the work of public health reformers who, in mid- to late nineteenth-century Britain, ensured that cities had proper sewers, clean water, and increasingly safe food supplies (Szreter 1988).

As well as being wrong about steady increases in living standards in nineteenth-century Britain, McKeown provides no evidence that British diets improved during this time. He infers that they improved; however, as noted, this inference is based on faulty assumptions about steady improvements in the standard of living in the nineteenth century. While his argument that personal medical care was irrelevant to declines in mortality at this time remains valid, as his critics have demonstrated medical intervention (more broadly defined as enhancements in the public health infrastructure) was likely important for health status advances in the general population (Szreter 1988).

In spite of the differences in Apple's and McKeown's approaches to historical questions regarding the social determinants of health, and in spite of the different nations and eras they investigated, they share the central hypothesis that better feeding of the population mediated the impact of economic change on health. The purpose of this and the next chapter is to explore this general thesis. However, while they investigated their hypotheses during what they believed were times of economic growth, this central hypothesis is explored in relation to the economic dislocation of Depression-era Canada.

Two key questions arise from Apple's and McKeown's work. First, in spite of a decade of economic dislocation, could the quality, safety, and availability of food in the general population and, most important, among the poor and vulnerable, have improved? And second, in spite of severe economic distress, were there improvements in the public health infrastructure and did these contribute to the widespread general improvements in health status observed in Canada in the 1930s?

Public health advances could have improved health directly by upgrading sanitation infrastructure, leading to the wider availability of germ-free water and food. The combination of enhanced resistance to disease due to improved access to food and reduced exposure to pathogens due to public health improvements could have produced the better health status witnessed in the 1930s.

From a social determinants of health point of view, the improvement in health in Canada at this time is a paradox because investigations of the relationship between health status and the economy have found that economic deterioration is usually accompanied by declines in population health status (DHHS 1980; Hertzman et al. 1996; Heymann et al. 2005; Marmot et al. 1995; Wilkinson 1989, 1996). Were there special circumstances in 1930s Canada that buffered the impact of economic dislocation on health status? And were these related to food availability and/or improvements in public health infrastructure?

As well, the impact of the Depression on the generation that experienced it was profound. Public attitudes and policies related to nutrition and health in the quarter century following the Depression were formed in the crucible of the 1930s. This means that, in order to understand how nutrition policy evolved after the Second World War, it is crucial to understand how these issues were understood and addressed in the 1930s.

The first section of this chapter tests McKeown's and Apple's broad "improvement-in-feeding" thesis indirectly by determining changes in the price and supply of basic food items during the 1930s and, thus, obtaining data on the national food supply situation. The first dietary surveys of vulnerable urban families were conducted in Canada in the late 1930s. The second section discusses the results of these surveys, which, although limited, provide the first scientific information on the diets of low-income Canadians. The third section discusses how these surveys were interpreted at the time of their publication (in the late 1930s and early 1940s) and subsequently.

The Depression and Food Supply
National food disappearance data are calculated by adding the amount of food produced and imported during a year plus stocks available at the beginning of that year. The net supply (i.e., what is available for consumption) is determined by subtracting domestic stock, as well as food used in manufacturing and livestock feed and food that is exported, at the end of the year. The net supply is divided by the Canadian population on 1 July of a given year to determine per capita food availability for that year. While the use of national disappearance data results in an overestimation of food supplies available on a per-capita basis for domestic consumption, it does provide a reasonable picture of the changing supply of food over time.

Figures 7.2 and 7.3 show that the domestic supply of most staples, except pork (and, early in the Depression, eggs and beef), was either stable or had increased during the Depression. Pork may have been increasingly replaced by beef as the price of the latter, higher-status, food declined dramatically during the Depression and was marketed intensively by the federal Department of Agriculture (Department of Agriculture 1930-39).

Figure 7.2

Per capita domestic disappearance of meat and selected dairy products by year, 1926-39

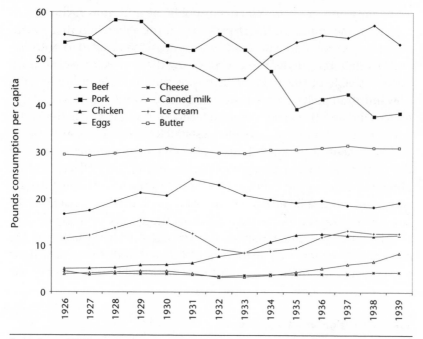

Source: Leacy (1993).

These data indicate that, at least at the national level, the supply of staple foods either remained stable or increased during the Depression.[2]

Surplus Food and Low Food Prices in the 1930s

In the 1930s relief programs involving direct food and cash distribution for unemployed families occurred within a deflationary economic environment. Even though wages fell across Canada by 14 percent between 1929 and 1933, there was a 22.5 percent decline in the cost of living during this time (Bliss 1987, 423). Bliss notes that, although by 1937 wages had climbed back to levels characteristic of the late 1920s (419),

---

[2] Given that export and import markets for agricultural produce were virtually closed during most of the 1930s, food disappearance data for this decade, compared to any other decade prior or since, provides an almost "pure" description of domestic food supply (i.e., based mainly on domestic production and consumption).

Figure 7.3

Per capita domestic disappearance of potatoes, wheat flour, milk, and total dairy products by year, 1926-39

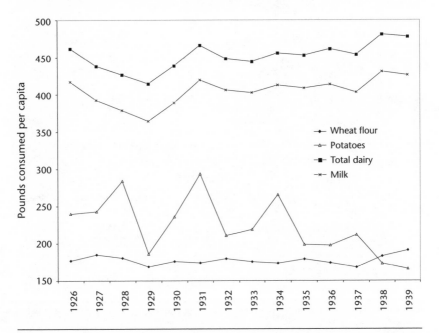

Source: Leacy (1993).

"most Canadians who kept their jobs during the depression enjoyed an improvement in their material, though not necessarily their psychic, standard of living" (423).

A major reason for the falling cost of living was continuing high domestic agricultural output combined with closed international agricultural markets, which depressed the price of Canadian food products. Figure 7.4 shows the price of selected staple food items in urban centres in Canada from 1914 to 1939. In the face of shortages, food prices rose during the First World War, peaking in 1920. During the early 1920s prices fell, stabilizing by the middle of the decade. After climbing briefly in the late 1920s, beginning in 1930 prices dropped, reaching their lowest level in 1933. Between 1933 and 1939 the price of key staples rose but only very slowly (Dominion Bureau of Statistics 1960).

On average, urban prices for key staples during the 1930s were less than they had been during the 1920s. Prices dropped 14 percent for milk and 39 percent for butter in the 1930s relative to the 1920s. In

Figure 7.4

Price of selected staple food items in urban Canada by year, 1914-39

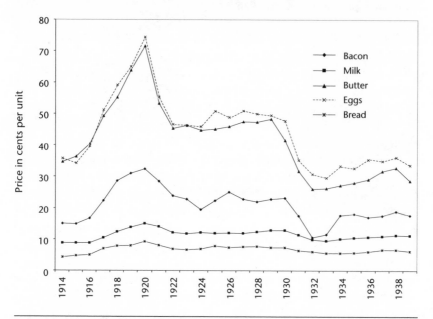

Note: For bacon, bread, and butter, prices are cents per pound; eggs are cents per dozen; milk is cents per quart.
Source: Dominion Bureau of Statistics (1960).

1933 the prices of butter, eggs, and bacon were less than they had been in 1914, and the prices for milk and bread were only marginally higher. As Figure 7.4 shows, throughout the Depression the prices of eggs and butter remained lower than prices in 1914. However, while this positive price and supply situation says something about the national structure of the urban food market in the 1930s, these data provide no information about food availability and security in cities in different regions of the country. And they tell us nothing about rural Canada.[3]

Is there any direct evidence that food supply improved in vulnerable regions or vulnerable subpopulations and that this led to either stable or better diets during the 1930s? The only way to directly obtain this type of information is to turn to dietary surveys. Modern dietary survey

---

[3]   Given that, at this time, 50 percent of the population lived in rural regions and that, outside drought-afflicted Saskatchewan and eastern Alberta, food production was high, the availability of food in rural Canada was probably fairly adequate.

methodology was developed in the early 1930s, and surveys of various subpopulations had been conducted in Britain (Boyd-Orr 1936) and the United States by 1935 (Stiebeling 1933). In Canada several dietary surveys had been conducted by 1939, mainly among low- and middle-income families (Department of Agriculture 1932; Hunter and Pett 1941; McHenry 1939; Patterson and McHenry 1941; Pett 1944; Pett and Hanley 1947; Sylvestre and Nadeau 1941; Young 1941). These surveys describe the diets mainly of low- and middle-income city dwellers, and they also provide insight into the early history of nutritional science in Canada.

Food Marketing Surveys in the 1930s
The earliest studies to assess the quality of the Canadian diet were marketing investigations conducted by the Department of Agriculture in order to better understand the impact of low income on the purchase of milk. The first of these, undertaken in 1931, was an analysis of milk marketing in Sydney, Glace Bay, and surrounding towns in Cape Breton in Nova Scotia. This study showed that "those in the higher income groups purchased the most milk per person, the average being 0.63 pints per day" (Department of Agriculture 1932, 86).

A second Department of Agriculture survey, conducted in 1935, studied 2,600 families living in Oshawa, Quebec, and Calgary; 251 families in villages near these three cities; and an additional 360 families living on farms outside these cities. Data on per-capita consumption of cheese, meat, eggs, and fish according to family income were obtained from the 2,600 families living in the cities (Canadian Preparatory Committee Report 1936, 79). Data on the per-capita consumption of *fresh* milk according to family income were obtained from this three-city survey as well as from the additional sample of 251 village and 360 farm families in the surrounding regions (see Figure 7.5) (ibid., 75).

These data show a regular gradient in which the consumption of protective foods steadily decreases, moving from high- to low-income families. Families earning more than $4,000 per year consumed 69 percent more fish, 43 percent more milk, 42 percent more meat, 34 percent more eggs, and 13 percent more cheese than did families on relief. These early marketing studies show that the poor ate less dairy products and meat than did the rich and that those on relief ate even less of these foods than did the poorest working families.

Although they showed that the availability of these traditionally expensive protective foods was related, in a regular gradient, with income (i.e., that as one moved up the income scale quantity and quality of food consumption steadily improved), the surveys tell us nothing about

Figure 7.5

Relative per capita consumption of various protective foods in 1935 in relation to family income

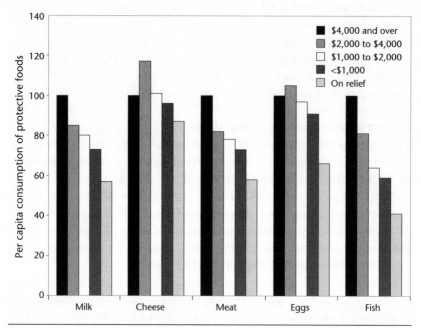

Note: The consumption value for families earning $4,000 or more annually is set at 100.
Source: Canadian Preparatory Committee of the British Commonwealth Scientific Conference (1936, 58-94).

the nutritional, physiological, or health status of individuals consuming these different diets. In other words, these studies demonstrate that the poor ate less well than did those with higher incomes, but they do not tell us whether the diets of the poor and unemployed on relief were adequate or whether these people suffered from undernourishment or malnourishment. In order to determine whether diets were adequate to maintain or improve health, new scientifically based dietary survey methods had to be developed, and the results of the application of these methods had to be compared with scientific standards of dietary adequacy.

Dietary Standards in the 1930s

A modern "dietary standard is a numerical expression, usually a daily average, of the quantities of certain nutrients believed to be needed by an individual representative of one of the various categories into which a population may be divided" (Young 1964, 302). A crude dietary standard was developed in Britain in 1862 and in Germany in the 1870s (Young 1964). In the United States similar standards were developed by Atwater and Bryant in the late nineteenth century and by Sherman in the first two decades of the twentieth century (Peterkin 1994). These were crude standards for adult males and females, establishing basal requirements for fat, protein, carbohydrate, and total energy.

The dietary standards developed in the nineteenth century were used to plan food production and distribution, usually for entire populations during such crises as crop failure or wartime mobilization. They were developed in laboratories during the course of feeding and feeding deprivation experiments on small numbers of test subjects as well as by nutrient intake surveys. With regard to the latter method, intake was usually measured over time among a small group of people who maintained their body weight so that a crude estimate of the nutrients and calories required to maintain normal physiological functioning and health could be determined. However, until the mid-twentieth century and the development of the first assay methods for measuring vitamins and minerals in blood and urine, dietary standards were relatively crude and were available mainly for fat, protein, carbohydrate, and total energy.

In the mid-1930s methods for developing dietary standards were improved upon in three ways. First, in recognition of the fact that people of different gender and ages have different nutrient requirements, standards were developed separately for men and women and for children of different genders and ages. Second, they were further modified by assessing the nutrient requirements for people engaged in various levels of physical exertion and for lactating and pregnant women (Young 1964). And third, the first crude standards for vitamins were developed.[4]

The lead in developing new dietary standards was taken by the League of Nations and was based largely on the scientific work conducted by John Boyd-Orr in England and Harriet Stiebeling in the United States. By the mid-1930s the League of Nations, the United States Department of Agriculture, and the British Medical Association had developed new dietary standards, including standards for vitamins (Young 1964). And in Canada the Ontario Medical Association, borrowing heavily from the British Medical Association, also developed a dietary standard specifically for families on unemployment relief (see Chapter 9).

---

[4] After the Second World War further refinements were made. In particular, standards were developed for girls, boys, and adult females and males of different heights and weights.

In the mid-1930s both Boyd-Orr and Stiebeling began to use these improved dietary standards in a new way – to judge the adequacy of diets that were measured using modern dietary survey methods. These surveys utilized detailed audits, usually of non-representative samples, to measure food intake either for families or for individuals within families. Once measured in this way food intake was converted, using food composition tables, to daily nutrient and energy intakes for entire families and/or individuals within families. These values were then compared with dietary standards in order to determine the adequacy of the diets being measured.

In the mid-1930s the League of Nations encouraged member countries both to conduct dietary surveys and to develop modern national dietary standards in order to scientifically assess the nutritional status of their populations. In 1938 Canada was the first nation in the world to establish a modern national dietary standard. It was this standard that nutrition scientists used to gauge the adequacy of the diets measured in the few dietary surveys that were conducted in Canada as the Depression finally began to ease in the late 1930s.

Dietary Surveys in Canada in the 1930s

In 1937/38 a survey of middle- and low-income Torontonians was conducted. This first dietary survey was organized by the Toronto Welfare Council and was conducted with the expert help of Dr. E.W. McHenry, one of Canada's leading nutritionists (McHenry 1939). In 1939 four more dietary surveys were conducted among middle- and low-income families in Edmonton (Hunter and Pett 1941), Halifax (Young 1941), Quebec City (Sylvestre and Nadeau 1941), and (again) Toronto (Patterson and McHenry 1941).

None of these surveys was conducted with unemployed people on relief: all were conducted with low- and middle-income working families. The surveys were usually based on non-random samples of urban families, which usually consisted, in English Canada, of people of "British" descent and, in Quebec City, of people of "French" descent. None of these surveys was conducted in rural regions or among urban immigrants or Aboriginal peoples.

The methods used in all five surveys relied on seven-day audits of family food expenditures as well as on direct measurements of individual food intakes, which were undertaken by weighing the food consumed by each individual in each family. Food intakes measured in this way were converted to values for energy and nutrient intake using food composition tables developed in the late 1930s by Canadian biochemists and nutritionists (Pett 1942).[5]

The five surveys conducted in Canadian cities in the late 1930s were small. Sample sizes ranged from approximately 300 to 600 individuals. In the Quebec City survey, average family income was $1,115 per annum, with a range from $600 to $1,500. Among these families, 40 percent of income was spent on food (Sylvestre and Nadeau 1941). In the 1937/38 Toronto survey, average family income was $1,021 per annum, with a range of from $520 to $1,820 equally distributed on either side of the average (McHenry 1939). In the second Toronto survey, conducted in 1939, average family income was $1,984 per annum, with a range from $1,300 to $3,250 equally distributed on either side of the average (Patterson and McHenry 1941). Average family incomes in both the Edmonton and the Halifax surveys were approximately $1,000 per annum, with a range from $450 to $1,500 equally distributed on either side of the average. In the Edmonton and Halifax surveys, 30 percent to 60 percent of family income was spent on food (Hunter and Pett 1941; Young 1941).

[5] Most subsequent large-scale dietary surveys have been conducted using the twenty-four-hour recall method. These early surveys, conducted with seven-day direct audits of food consumption, may have obtained more precise estimates than are obtained in today's dietary surveys as direct week-long assessments of food consumption "smooth out" the variation in daily intakes, resulting in more accurate estimates of an individual's food consumption. As well, weighing of amounts consumed by each individual obtains much more accurate measures of intake than modern recall methods. Comparisons between dietary surveys based on seven-day measures of food consumption and a dietary standards is more statistically valid than are comparisons between dietary surveys based on twenty-four-hour recall and dietary standards (Beaton 1981). The greater statistical validity of methods used in the 1930s is due to the fact that, in measuring consumption over seven days, individual variability in food intake is better measured than it is with twenty-four hour recall. However, the early surveys were usually conducted with convenience samples rather than with representative samples, from which generalizations about the dietary status of larger populations could be accurately made. As well, because it is difficult to obtain information on the quality of the supervision of field workers in these studies, it is impossible to gauge the accuracy of measurements of food consumption. Finally, the Canadian food composition tables, which converted measured food intake to vitamin and micro-nutrient intakes, were only developed in the late 1930s. They were somewhat crude, so that the accuracy of the translation of consumed food into values for vitamin and micro-nutrient intake is impossible to ascertain.

Given that the methods used in the five surveys were roughly similar (i.e., one week of directly measuring food consumed by individuals), the average energy and nutrient intakes measured can be compared with each other to produce a rough picture of food consumption in low-income families in some Canadian cities in the late 1930s. And average values for energy and nutrient levels obtained in these studies can be compared with the 1938 basal national standard to determine, again in rough fashion, the adequacy of diets, at least according to the standards of the 1930s, among all survey respondents.

The results for four of the five surveys conducted in the late 1930s are found in Table 7.1. This table also shows the average results across the four surveys, the 1938 standard for energy and some nutrients, and the percentage difference between this standard and the averaged results of the four surveys.[6]

For males, in three of the four surveys conducted in 1938, energy intake was greater than the Canadian standard. For females, in 1938 in three of the four surveys energy intake was slightly below the standard. Averaging results across the four dietary surveys and comparing these to the 1938 standard demonstrates that mean energy intake for males was 4.8 percent higher than the standard, while for females it was 5.7 percent lower.

For both men and women, protein intake in three of the four surveys was greater than the standard. Averaging the results of the four dietary surveys and comparing these to the standard demonstrates that the mean protein intake for males was 14.9 percent higher than the standard, while that for females was 1.2 percent lower. Average fat intake, available in only two of the four surveys, was greater than the standard for both genders. For men, mean calcium levels across the four surveys were approximately 12 percent greater than the standard, while for women they were approximately 12 percent lower. For men, iron levels were slightly below the standard; for women, they were approximately one-quarter less than the standard.

Finally, two of the surveys (Patterson & McHenry, 1941; Young, 1941) published vitamin results which showed, per respondent, intakes of vitamin B were from 42 to 69 percent of the 1938 standard and for Vitamin C they ranged from 59 to 90 percent of the standard. The other two surveys did not report vitamin results but stated that they were also below standard for vitamins B and C.

---

[6] Results for the Edmonton survey are not shown as these were expressed as family averages and are therefore not easily compared with the results of the other surveys, which present results for each individual in the family.

Table 7.1

Results from four Canadian dietary surveys conducted in the 1930s in relation to the 1938 dietary standard for males and females

	Males					Females				
	Calories	Protein* (g)	Fat (g)	Ca+ (g)	Fe+ (mg)	Calories	Protein* (g)	Fat (g)	Ca+ (g)	Fe+ (mg)
Halifax (Young 1941)	2,622	95.0	120.0	0.60	15.0	1,963	68.0	89.0	0.46	12.0
Toronto (McHenry 1939)	2,360	60.2	N/A*	0.64	11.5	1,720	40.9	N/A*	0.49	8.0
Toronto (Patterson & McHenry 1941)	2,540	82.0	102.0	0.83	13.7	1,930	61.0	78.0	0.65	10.6
Edmonton (Hunter & Pett 1941)	2,539	84.4	N/A*	0.59	17.7	1,932	59.4	N/A*	0.51	13.9
Four-survey average	2,515	80.4	111.0	0.67	14.5	1,886	57.3	83.5	0.53	11.1
1938 basal standard	2,400	70.0	85.0	0.60	15.0	2,000	58.0	77	0.60	15.0
% difference between survey average and 1938 standard	4.8	14.9	15.4	11.7	-3.3	-5.7	-1.2	8.4	-11.7	-26.0

* Fat intake was not measured in the Toronto (McHenry 1939) and Edmonton (Hunter and Pett 1941) surveys.

Sources: These data are derived from four surveys. Two were conducted in Toronto (McHenry 1939; Patterson and McHenry 1941), one was conducted in Edmonton (Hunter and Pett 1941), and the fourth survey was conducted in Halifax (Young 1941).

Controversy over the Dietary Surveys

In the spring of 1939 the results of the first Toronto dietary survey, sponsored by the Toronto Welfare Council with E.W. McHenry's expert guidance, were published. In summing up the results of this survey, McHenry (1939, 9) opined that "on the whole the men did reasonably well but one is forced to conclude that the women and children were inadequately nourished." He also roughly divided this sample of low-income Toronto families into the highest- and lowest-income groups. Comparing the energy, protein, calcium, and iron intakes across these groups he found minimal difference. Based mainly on this comparison, he concluded that low income was not a barrier to obtaining an adequate diet and that better use of existing monies would solve the problem of dietary inadequacy. In particular, he advised that "mothers should be given training in the essential principles of nutrition and purchasing" (11).

However, the Toronto Welfare Council concluded from the survey that there is "evidence of harm resulting from the low standard of living made necessary by inadequate income" (quoted in Struthers 1991, 70). It used the survey results to campaign hard for an increase in relief rates; however, this was to no avail as in 1939 the Ontario government proceeded to cut relief rates in Toronto's suburbs.

The attitude of other nutrition scientists conducting dietary surveys in Toronto, Edmonton, and Halifax at this time was not dissimilar to McHenry's. Patterson and McHenry (1941, 265), reporting on the second Toronto dietary survey, pointed "to the need for educational work giving information about nutritive values in relation to food cost. Especially great is this need among families with low purchasing power. An increasing amount of evidence shows clearly that many families are spending sufficient money to secure an adequate diet but are failing to do so because of a lack of knowledge regarding economical purchasing." And, commenting on their Edmonton survey, Hunter and Pett (1941, 265) concluded that "the only means left to try to maintain the health of the population – in so far as that is possible by adequate diets – is to teach people to make the most of their available money."

In academic papers based on these dietary surveys, the authors agreed that caloric intakes were adequate for men but not for women and that, relative to the dietary standard, the dietary intakes of most vitamins, calcium, and iron were too low for women. Given that these surveys were of the working poor and did not include families on relief, leading Canadian nutrition scientists were fairly certain that many members of low-income and unemployed families, particularly women and children, were suffering from vitamin and mineral deficiencies. Despite this concern, and knowing that they had no information on the diets of the unemployed, they were hesitant to advocate for increases in the food allowance for the unemployed.

Canadian nutritionists interpreted the results emerging from dietary surveys in the late 1930s in ways that did not place undue pressure on relief administrations; rather, they shifted responsibility for obtaining adequate nutrition from the state to mothers in low-income and unemployed households. This position, which was taken by most leading Canadian nutrition scientists, was also common among American nutritionists (Levenstein 1993).

Were the Poor and Unemployed Undernourished According to Modern Standards?

As outlined previously, the methods used in conducting dietary surveys in the 1930s, and today, as well as the standards themselves, were quite different so that simple comparison of results of these surveys with modern standards is difficult. When dietary surveys were first conducted in Britain, the United States, and Canada in the mid-1930s and reported on in the late 1930s and early 1940s, scientific problems with vitamin standards and methods of comparison between surveys and standards – and the interpretation and meaning of these comparisons – were not well understood. Many nutritionists were also uneasy with the high level of scientific uncertainty and unreliability in conducting vitamin assays and utilizing crude biochemical tables to convert food into energy and nutrient intakes. As Young (1941, 239) pointed out in discussing his Halifax survey, vitamins "present the most difficult results of the survey from which to draw sound conclusions. Methods of assay are open to large errors and human requirements are still uncertain." Commenting on the large proportion of adults with vitamin deficiency in the Halifax survey, he further commented that "this result may mean a serious deficiency in the Maritime food consumption or it may mean a standard that is too high" (ibid.).

In the post-Second World War decades, leading nutritionists in Canada gained a better understanding of the methodological problems of using dietary surveys in relation to dietary standards in order to predict "adequacy" of diets (Pett et al. 1945). For example, in discussing the methods and results of John Boyd-Orr's 1930s dietary surveys in Britain – some thirty years later and with the benefit of three decades of improvements in nutritional science – leading Canadian nutrition scientist Gordon Young (1964, 324) commented:

The danger of misuse of standards is well illustrated by Orr in his book entitled *Food, Health, and Income*, in which he drew the sweeping conclusion that in the United Kingdom the average diet of the poorest group of 4.5 million people was deficient in every dietary essential listed. Even in the wealthiest group, which included only 10 percent of the population, complete adequacy was not attained by the standard used. Likewise it was on a false basis of comparison that the dietary surveys in Canada in 1939 led to the conclusion of extensive dietary deficiencies. Against such conclusions were the astonishingly low statistics of mortality and morbidity for the deficiency diseases.

As well as the unreliability of vitamin measurement science, the standards for most vitamins and minerals (except for calcium) tended to be higher in 1938 than today. The 1938 standard for Vitamin C is similar to today's standards. However, the 1938 standard for protein, iron, and some vitamins (i.e., Vitamins D and A) (Health and Welfare Canada 1990; McHenry 1941b) was much higher than the standards we have now. While this in part may be because physical demands, particularly related to work, are much lower now than they were in the 1930s (and these lower demands are to some extent, and for some nutrients, related to lower standards), in general, the standards are lower today because they are based on more accurate methods of vitamin chemistry and a better understanding of the role of vitamins in human physiology.

In spite of the difficulties in comparing these 1930s dietary surveys with today's standards, a modern nutritionist would likely find that these late Depression-era diets were of poor quality, marked by too low a proportion of energy obtained from protein and too high a proportion obtained from fat. While iron intakes likely would be deemed as adequate, calcium intakes would be considered very low, especially for women. Like their 1930s counterparts, modern nutritionists would find the energy intakes for women slightly inadequate, and would also argue that the energy intakes for men were quite inadequate.

Summary
In 1930s Canada the national food supply likely did not deteriorate in spite of an extended period of economic crisis. Food production remained very high and food prices very low. The cost of living generally declined so that, for people with income, food availability was ensured. In most rural areas (at least outside drought-ravaged Saskatchewan – where the federal government intervened most aggressively to supply aid), and in

cities in which people had access to gardens, basic food supply may have been adequate.

These crude national price and supply data say nothing about hunger or malnutrition in vulnerable populations or in different regions of the country. For urban working men assessed in several dietary surveys conducted between 1937 and 1939, in comparison with the 1938 basal standard, there is no evidence that energy, vitamin, mineral, and protein intakes were inadequate. However, in reference to the 1938 basal standard, these surveys did show evidence of some energy deficiency and fairly extensive vitamin and mineral (especially calcium) deficiency among women and children. For the unemployed there is no information, except for a 1934 marketing survey that showed that both the working poor and the unemployed ate less well than did middle-income people; however, the survey could not be used to ascertain whether or not diets among these people were adequate. As well, these dietary surveys showed that men in poor families were the most well fed followed by children, and that mothers may have been cutting back on their own food consumption to ensure that these other family members were more adequately fed.

The results of these surveys were interpreted quite differently by community and advocacy groups, on the one hand, and the nutrition scientists who conducted them, on the other. Although both groups felt that the evidence pointed to vitamin and mineral deficiencies (among poor women and children), the community and advocacy groups called for increasing the food allowance as part of unemployment relief, while the nutritionists blamed mothers for making poor food purchasing, cooking, menu, and food storage choices. The nutritionist scientists recommended educating mothers in poor and unemployed families to improve diets.

These early dietary surveys were restricted to small urban samples and did not include families on relief, although they did include very low-income families. They were conducted when the country was emerging from the Depression, so their results do not reflect conditions experienced during its worst years. Also, the surveys included no rural families and very few persons of non-French or British ancestry.

In hindsight, total energy intake observed in these surveys was likely too low, with the proportion of energy obtained from protein too low and from fat too high, indicating that the diets of low-income urban Canadians were poor. Family members consuming these diets for a long time might suffer from hunger and lose weight, particularly if physical demands were high. While the extent of calcium deficiency was probably not exaggerated, the extent of iron and vitamin deficiency was likely overstated at the time.

Also, the overall extent of clinical nutritional problems in the Canadian population at this time was dependent on the size of this vulnerable group and the extent to which it was "exposed" to poor diets for long periods of time. A key factor in determining the nutritional experience in these marginal families (particularly those who were landless residents of rural regions or living in cities and towns) was clearly the size of the relief incomes they obtained as a few more dollars and even cents obtained from relief could mean the difference between dietary adequacy and inadequacy.

In spite of the fact that many poor and unemployed people struggled to feed their families during the economic crisis of the 1930s, the numbers in these marginal groups and the length of their exposure to inadequate diets was mitigated by a combination of high supply and low food prices, increased private charity, growing (albeit reluctant) federal government involvement in providing unemployment relief and direct food aid, and the pressure exerted on all levels of government by the unemployed and their allies.

8
Mortality from Nutritional Deficiency Diseases during the Depression

As Gordon Young (1964, 324) noted in the 1960s, while the Depression was a time of hunger for many, and while it was widely believed that malnutrition was widespread, the entire decade was characterized by "astonishingly low statistics of mortality and morbidity for the deficiency diseases."

This chapter outlines mortality trends due to nutritional deficiency diseases (i.e., rickets, scurvy, beriberi, osteomalacia, and pellagra). Morbidity from nutritional diseases would be a much better indicator of the extent of malnutrition and a more sensitive measure of its impact on health than mortality. However, morbidity data on nutritional diseases are not available for the 1930s. While the mortality data provide a relatively insensitive measure of the extent of malnutrition, it is likely that increases in nutritional deficiency disease, arising from decreasing food availability, would have been matched to some extent by increases in mortality from these diseases. Also, declines in mortality would likely have been matched by declines in the burden of illness due to nutritional deficiency.

The first section of this chapter reviews 1930s mortality trends for nutritional deficiency diseases. The second section outlines mortality trends for rickets, which was the most common nutritional deficiency disease in Canada in the 1930s. The third section looks at possible reasons for the decline in rickets deaths in relation to changes in food supply and public health reform. The fourth section discusses this evidence in relation to the thesis that, in spite of the prolonged economic crisis, better nutrition may have been partly responsible for improving the health status of the general population during the Depression.

Mortality from Nutritional Deficiency Diseases
In Canada, between 1926 and 1939, 1,856 deaths were recorded for nutritional deficiency disease (Dominion Bureau of Statistics 1921-51).

Approximately half of these 1,856 nutritional deficiency deaths occurred in the four years prior to the Depression (1926 to 1929) – a time when the economy was doing relatively well – while the other half occurred over a ten-year period (1930 to 1939) that was riven with economic crisis.

By far the most prevalent nutritional deficiency disease was rickets, accounting for 86.1 percent of such deaths over this period (Table 8.1). This was a disease mainly of children under the age of one year, and, as outlined in Chapter 4, was mainly due to a deficiency of Vitamin D. The next most prevalent nutritional deficiency disease at this time was scurvy, also often a disease of childhood. Finally, beriberi, osteomalacia, and pellagra also occurred (albeit rarely) during the 1930s (Table 8.2).

There are two points that arise from a review of non-rickets nutritional deficiency deaths in the 1930s. First, as is shown in Table 8.2, non-rickets deficiency deaths were extremely rare and relatively constant through the 1930s. If malnutrition was widespread, severe, and deepening as the Depression continued, particularly in vulnerable subpopulations, one would expect to see increases in mortality from these non-rickets nutritional deficiency diseases during this decade. As well, if malnutrition decreased markedly, then one would expect to see

Table 8.1

Number of deaths from rickets by region and by year, 1926-39

Year	Maritimes	Quebec	Ontario	Prairies	BC	Total	Percent
1926	13	117	51	24	6	211	12.8
1927	13	115	30	27	4	189	11.5
1928	7	124	51	38	2	222	13.5
1929	11	117	40	34	1	203	12.4
1930	21	95	49	32	3	200	12.2
1931	5	48	24	20	5	102	6.2
1932	10	49	19	14	3	95	5.8
1933	4	30	18	13	1	66	4.0
1934	4	36	17	11	4	72	4.4
1935	4	32	8	7	0	51	3.1
1936	6	32	12	16	2	68	4.1
1937	3	31	9	11	0	54	3.3
1938	7	22	15	14	3	61	3.7
1939	5	26	8	9	1	49	3.0
Total	113	874	351	270	35	1643	100
Percent	6.8	53.3	21.4	16.4	2.1	100	100

Source: Dominion Bureau of Statistics (1921-50).

Table 8.2

Number of deaths from non-rickets nutritional deficiency diseases by region and by year, 1926-39

Year	Maritimes	Quebec	Ontario	Prairies	BC	Total	Percent
1926	2	10	11	4	1	28	12.4
1927	0	5	3	1	1	10	4.4
1928	1	0	7	0	0	8	3.5
1929	0	3	9	1	2	15	6.6
1930	1	5	3	1	0	10	4.4
1931	1	6	5	2	0	14	6.2
1932	1	9	4	2	1	17	7.5
1933	1	5	8	1	1	16	7.1
1934	1	3	4	2	1	11	4.9
1935	1	10	5	2	3	21	9.3
1936	4	10	2	4	0	20	8.9
1937	1	5	2	6	1	15	6.6
1938	1	8	3	5	1	18	8.0
1939	1	9	8	2	3	23	10.2
Total	16	88	74	33	15	226	100
Percent	7.1	38.9	32.7	14.6	6.6	100	

Source: Dominion Bureau of Statistics (1921-50).

decreases in mortality from these illnesses. The fact that these deaths were rare and stable through the 1930s indicates that it is likely that a major deterioration in food availability to the most vulnerable segments of the population did not occur during the Depression. Furthermore, because the death rates from these diseases were higher in the four years prior to the Depression (1926-29), there is some evidence that the nutritional status of these groups likely improved during the Depression.

Why Did Rickets Mortality Decline in the 1930s?
Most nutritional deficiency deaths in the 1930s were due to rickets. Unlike deaths from non-rickets diseases, deaths from rickets plummeted during the Depression, declining by 71 percent from approximately 90 per 100,000 live births in the period between 1926 and 1929 to approximately 25 in the period between 1935 and 1939. This overall decline in the 1930s was driven by the dramatic lowering of rickets mortality among infants, particularly in Quebec (Figure 8.1).

Improvements in rickets mortality were likely driven by a combination of direct improvements in food access (in spite of rapidly declining breastfeeding rates), drastic declines in fertility, and enhancements in

Figure 8.1

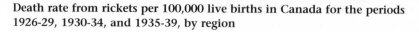

Death rate from rickets per 100,000 live births in Canada for the periods 1926-29, 1930-34, and 1935-39, by region

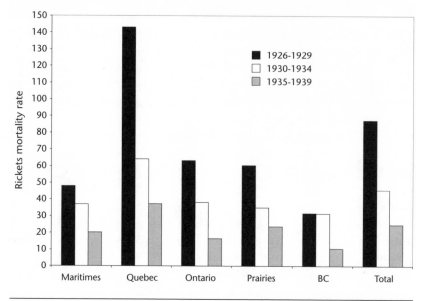

Note: The rickets mortality rate was calculated by summing deaths from rickets within each of the three time periods (1926-29, 1930-34, and 1935-39) and each of the five regions and dividing these by the number of live births in each time period. Infant mortality rates are usually expressed per 1,000 live births. Given the relative rarity of rickets deaths, these rates were expressed per 100,000 live births. The Maritimes region consists of Nova Scotia, New Brunswick, and PEI. The prairie region consists of Alberta, Saskatchewan, and Manitoba. *Sources:* live births by province: Dominion Bureau of Statistics (1926-39); total rickets deaths: Dominion Bureau of Statistics (1921-50).

public health education and infrastructure (especially those leading to improvements in food safety), particularly in Quebec.

With regard to improvements in food access, among a population of women who mainly breastfed their babies this could indirectly reduce rickets mortality because improved maternal nutrition would produce higher-quality breast milk (particularly in terms of Vitamin D and calcium) and, by improving maternal stamina, have the potential to increase the duration of breastfeeding. However, breastfeeding rates in Canada were dropping, and in Quebec at this time they were by far the lowest in the country (Chandler 1929; Thornton and Olson 1991, 1997, 2001). Thus enhanced feeding of mothers would not likely have had a direct impact on rickets mortality, especially in Quebec, where such improvements were most dramatic.

Another explanation may be that the dissemination of anti-rickets advice, beginning in 1926 through *The Canadian Mother's Book*, was successful. At the time the *CMB* also advised mothers to breastfeed and, while this advice was being increasingly by-passed in favour of artificial feeding, it is possible that, by the early 1930s, increasing numbers of Canadian women were beginning to unswaddle their babies, expose them to the sun, and feed them cod-liver oil.

Poor mothers may have consumed similar, or even worse, diets than did more affluent mothers as economic conditions deteriorated in the 1930s, but by feeding their babies cod-liver oil and/or exposing them to more sunlight, they may have managed to stave off rickets. Of course, it would be necessary to have evidence that poor and vulnerable families (particularly those residing in rural Quebec) received the *CMB* or similar information regularly and, second, that they acted on its anti-rickets advice.

It's not clear to what extent mothers in poor households received the *CMB*, although we know it was widely distributed for much of the 1930s (including in French and in Quebec). However, we do know that increased contact between pregnant women and new mothers and the medical profession occurred across Canada as birthing was increasingly hospitalized. And, with the expansion of the public health infrastructure, it is likely that the increasing interaction between mothers and physicians resulted in the increased dissemination of advice on supplementing infant feeding with cod-liver oil.

The decline in rickets mortality may also have been due to general improvements in the public health infrastructure particularly those resulting in improved availability of clean water and cow's milk. In Quebec the provincial public health system was reorganized in 1922, a campaign against tuberculosis and infant mortality was initiated, and twenty municipalities constructed filtration systems to purify their water as rural areas began to clean up local water supplies (Anctil 1986). In 1926 "unités sanitaires" were created, and the responsibility for these units was transferred from municipalities to the province.

A major typhoid epidemic, due to contaminated milk, broke out in Montreal in 1927. Provincial medical health officers pressured the province to make milk pasteurization mandatory. The Montreal typhoid epidemic was a watershed, and, throughout the 1930s, it created great momentum for pasteurizing milk not only in the city and but also throughout the province (Anctil and Bluteau 1986).

In 1933 further legislation was passed to better finance medical health units throughout Quebec. Clinics were formed for the care and

Figure 8.2

Infant mortality per 1,000 live births by year and region in Canada, 1921-45

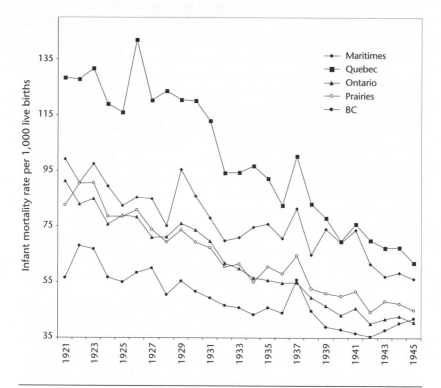

Source: Statistics Canada (1991, Table 2b, 34).

prevention of tuberculosis and for the care of newborns in both urban and rural regions of the province (Anctil and Bluteau 1986). The public health infrastructure in rural Quebec, as well as in other rural regions of Canada, was in fact upgraded significantly and may have played an important role in the dramatic declines in infant mortality observed throughout the 1930s (Figure 8.2).

As shown in Figure 8.2, there was a general decline in infant mortality across Canada in the 1930s. This is yet more evidence that the social (including nutritional) conditions for families with infants improved across Canada at this time. While the dissemination of targeted anti-rickets advice may have contributed to the decline in infant deaths due to rickets, the generalized decline indicates that broader forces were in play across Canada.[1]

As is well known, an increased spacing between births tends to improve the survival chances of children, probably because mothers are less overworked and, with less competition, each infant has a better chance of obtaining the nourishment needed to survive (Bideau et al. 1997). In other words, more spacing, assuming a stable family food supply, increases the availability of food for each surviving infant.

Declines in birth rates in the 1930s led to increased spacing between births, which, in turn, led to increased food availability per infant. And this occurred within the context of some improvement in water and milk supplies, particularly in Quebec.[2]

Revisiting Apple's and McKeown's Hypothesis

The previous chapter began by asking why the health of citizens in general, and infants in particular, improved so dramatically during this long decade of economic hardship? The past two chapters have explored the idea, first developed by McKeown, that access to food mediates the relationship between economic change and health status.

---

[1] In the 1920s, the difference in infant mortality between British Columbia and Quebec was astounding. In today's terms, this would be as though British Columbia had current Canadian infant mortality rates (about 5 deaths per 1,000 live births) and as though Quebec had rates typical of a third-world country such as Jamaica. While in 1921 this was an extreme comparison (healthiest province with unhealthiest province), the infant mortality rate in Quebec was still 45 percent higher than that of its neighbour, Ontario. These regional differences in infant mortality, at a time when most deaths were due to infectious disease, indicate that social and economic conditions in Quebec were much worse than they were in the rest of Canada and that this was a very underdeveloped part of the country. The difference in infant morality rates in Quebec and British Columbia was "only" 200 percent by 1939, indicating some narrowing. Figure 8.2 shows that, besides Quebec, the other big "winner" in the decline in infant mortality during the Depression was Ontario, which in 1921 had infant morality rates that were approximately 50 percent higher than those in British Columbia. By 1939 BC rates and Ontario rates were similar, and in 1945 they were the same (and the lowest in the country).

[2] There is another possible explanation that women, facing food shortages and poverty reverted increasingly to breastfeeding as the depression unfolded. There are no data from the 1930s on breastfeeding rates so this cannot be ruled out. However, the declines in both rickets and infant mortality were most dramatic in rural Quebec, where reversion to breastfeeding was highly unlikely given the cultural bias among French Canadian mothers against the practice.

There were several unique features to the agri-economic situation in Canada in the 1930s. For most of the decade agricultural production was high, food prices were historically low, and, during the most severe part of the Depression, prices declined faster than wages so that the cost of living for those who remained employed improved. In situations of economic trauma, where food is widely available and cheap, poor people do not have to find ever-increasing amounts of money to buy food. In other words inflation in food prices is not an issue. For rural landless people and poor people living in the towns and cities survival depends on finding direct food aid, a job, or income from relief or charity.

Infant mortality, including deaths from rickets, improved markedly in Canada during the Depression. According to most public health experts, rapid improvements in infant mortality, which occurred in developed nations at various times from the 1890s through the 1930s, were due mainly to improvements in the cleanliness of milk and water – particularly important environmental determinants of infant health as mothers abandoned breastfeeding (Rosen 1958).

While the federal system of food safety, through surveillance for adulteration, was involved in ensuring that dairy products were germ free, public health efforts to clean up the water and milk supplies were mainly initiated and financed by municipal and provincial governments. As outlined in previous chapters, these efforts were uneven both across and within regions in Canada, particularly in the 1930s as lower levels of government were increasingly short of cash.

Both Apple and McKeown postulated that rising standards of living led to increased access to food, which, in turn, led to better health (in Apple's case, among children in the early twentieth-century United States, and in McKeown's case, in the general population in nineteenth-century Britain). Both theses erred in relying on the assumption that economic conditions improved markedly during these times, and both assumed that improved health status was driven by better diets and, in Apple's case, more and better quality care by physicians.

However, there is some indirect, albeit crude, evidence in the form of trends in nutritional deficiency disease mortality, that under- and malnutrition was not widespread among vulnerable subpopulations in Canada during the 1930s. Deaths from non-rickets nutritional deficiency diseases remained extremely rare and constant even as the Depression deepened. And deaths from rickets declined dramatically in the 1930s. It is quite likely that declines in infant deaths were due to a relatively stable supply of cheap food in combination with public health infrastructural enhancement and increased birth spacing (particularly in Quebec, where declines both in infant and rickets mortality were most dramatic).[3]

Summary

The evidence from this and the previous chapter indicates that the 1930s, although extremely hard for many people, likely offered better access to food than did the 1920s and that, as the decade unfolded, food availability did not deteriorate. Thus, in spite of a lowered standard of living for a significant proportion of the population, it is possible that the wide availability of relatively cheap food, even among disadvantaged subgroups, in conjunction with improvements in public health infrastructure (particularly in rural regions) and increased birth spacing, could have contributed to the better health status among Canadians during the Depression than during the 1920s.

However, many people had difficulty adequately feeding their families and this greatly affected political developments. As is demonstrated in the next chapter, the massive social and political changes under way in the 1930s, in particular the financial breakdown of municipal and provincial governments, initiated a historically unprecedented use of the federal government's constitutionally sanctioned spending power in the arena of both health and social policy. This led directly to the formation of the Canadian Council on Nutrition, the first agency created specifically to advise the government on nutrition policy. It is to these developments that I now turn.

---

[3] Improvements in public health infrastructure, which led to cleaner cow's milk and water, were in fact the result of enhancements of food safety.

9

The Canadian Council on Nutrition and the First National Dietary Standard

Until the late 1940s, dietary standards were developed by governments in response to food shortages due to war, agricultural failures, and/or distribution problems arising from economic and political crises (Leitch 1942). In 1862 the British government, in response to an agricultural crisis and related civil unrest, developed the world's first dietary standard, which was designed to avert starvation and disease among the poor and destitute (Smith 1863). A second dietary standard was developed by the British towards the end of the First World War, again in response to potential food shortages (Lusk 1918). This became the first national dietary standard ever established (Leitch 1942).

The economic crisis of the 1930s spurred the next round of dietary standard-setting. A committee of the British Medical Association established a dietary standard in 1933. In the same year, in the United States, Hazel Stiebeling, working in the Department of Agriculture, established a standard to maintain optimal health, incorporating the latest vitamin discoveries (Smith 2000; Stiebeling 1933). Then, in 1935, the League of Nations developed an international dietary standard whose main purpose was both to improve national diets and to restimulate agricultural production and international trade (League of Nations 1936). Several German standards were also developed in the nineteenth century (Peterkin 1994).

In Canada, two years prior to publication of the League's standard, the Ontario Medical Association (OMA) established a dietary standard for families receiving social assistance, which, in the mid-1930s, was used by some municipal and provincial welfare administrations in that province to determine social assistance rates (OMA 1933). The Canadian government moved quickly to endorse the OMA relief standard and to establish both a national nutrition policy-making organization –

the Canadian Council on Nutrition (CCN) – and, in the spring of 1938, a Canadian national dietary standard (CCN 1938a).

Widely publicized vitamin discoveries, new metabolic studies, and more sophisticated and comprehensive dietary survey methods had, during the interwar years, increased the effectiveness and status of nutrition science in both lay and scientific circles (Smith 2000). The 1933 Stiebeling standard established requirements for a number of minerals and vitamins, representing the first major scientific improvement in dietary standards since the original British standard, which had been established approximately seventy years earlier.

As the Depression deepened, the League of Nations promoted research, disseminated the new nutrition science, and actively fostered the establishment of nutrition policy-making institutions. The League saw the adoption of national dietary standards as central to an international economic strategy to break the Depression's stranglehold. It felt that, if nations developed scientifically authoritative dietary standards, and if they established new national nutritional policy-making institutions to improve research and awareness of dietary inadequacy, then the quality and quantity of national diets could be improved. This would create more demand for food, which in turn, would increase worldwide agricultural production, thus restimulating international trade and ending the economic crisis.

The purpose of this chapter is to describe the social and political conditions leading both to the establishment of the Canadian Council on Nutrition and the national dietary standard. The first section begins by discussing the problem of unemployment in the 1930s in relation to emerging dietary standards. The second section outlines domestic and international policy developments in relation to unemployment and dietary standards. The third section discusses the policy developments that led to the establishment of the first dietary standard and the formation of the CCN in relation to the results of the 1930s dietary surveys. The final section outlines the scientific and policy position taken by most of Canada's nutrition scientists as they developed the national dietary standard.

Unemployment and Dietary Standards

By 1933 the mushrooming cost of relief payments left many municipalities and provinces near bankruptcy (Saunders and Back 1940). Provinces were constitutionally responsible for providing unemployment relief – setting standards for eligibility and rates for relief payments – but in practice this was often downloaded to local municipalities, who paid for relief mainly through property taxes. The deep and sustained unemployment overwhelmed municipal and provincial governments, triggering limited federal intervention in the form of loans and cash grants (Canada 1954). By 1936 this situation was increasingly untenable because the federal government had no constitutional authority over unemployment relief assistance and, therefore, no control over relief costs. Yet it was paying most of the national relief bill.

By the mid-1930s the federal government began to impose standards for relief administration as a condition for cash grants and loans to the provinces (Saunders and Back 1940). As the unemployment crisis deepened in 1937, the National Employment Commission advised that, in order to improve labour mobility and productivity as well as the efficiency of relief spending, the federal government should develop an integrated national system of employment training, placement, and unemployment insurance (Struthers 1983).

Part of the rationale for implementing such a system was to standardize and control the costs of relief administration by improving its efficiency (Struthers 1983). The 1938 Royal Commission on Federal-Provincial Relations reflected the prevailing government view: "The deficiency of relief food allowances in body building proteins and protective foods is bound to have bad effects on families who must live on them for long periods of time. Undermining of physique and destruction of morale are then inevitable. The state must later pay the permanent costs of unemployability, illness, crime, and immorality. The lack of standards in relief administration has injured the taxpayer and continues to do so" (Grauer 1939, 24).

Thus, the federal government, at least outside the health department, had little understanding of, or interest in, the relationship between long-term food deprivation and health – and then, in classic utilitarian fashion, the concern was about potential impacts on finances. Government was interested in streamlining national unemployment relief administration, and, although concerns were mounting about hunger and its possible impacts on health among reform-minded physicians and citizens' groups, this was not a major consideration for federal government policy makers.

As the Depression deepened, municipal and provincial governments were pressured by left-wing political and community groups, and organizations of unemployed workers, to expand relief programs and to offer more generous assistance. Because of the high proportion of relief incomes spent on food, debates about appropriate relief rates coalesced around the quality and quantity of food required to sustain the health of families receiving cash assistance.[1] At the same time, the League of Nations was aggressively promoting nutrition science as the key to solving the global unemployment crisis.

It was this pressure from the League of Nations that led Canada (albeit for different reasons than those envisioned by the League) to establish national nutrition policy-making institutions. Before turning to these developments it is important to describe the domestic nutrition policy-making situation in Canada in the early and mid-1930s.

Domestic Stakeholders and Policy Makers

Both the Canadian Medical Association and the Ontario Medical Association formed nutrition committees that worked fairly closely with community groups concerned with health conditions among the growing army of unemployed workers and their families.[2] Activist groups were also involved. In Toronto, for example, women's organizations and child welfare and dieticians' organizations such as the Visiting Homemaker's Association were particularly active in the mid-1930s in pressuring welfare administrators to increase relief rates (McReady 1934).

In Ontario, early in the Depression, when the provincial government moved to standardize the administration of unemployment relief, debate centred on the proportion of the relief allowance to be spent on food (Campbell 1932). The focus of the debates was money – that is, the government's ability to pay – but there was little scientific information available on the quality or quantity of food required to maintain health. This changed in 1933 when the Ontario Medical Association published a dietary standard based on Stiebeling's American standard (OMA 1933) (Table 9.1). The OMA translated its dietary standard into typical Canadian family diets and then priced these, demonstrating that the cost of

---

[1] In September 1936 the proportion of relief allowances spent for food ranged from a low of 44 percent in Hull, Quebec, to a high of 77 percent in Victoria, British Columbia (Struthers 1983, 212).

[2] In Ontario in 1932 a limited health insurance plan for people receiving unemployment benefits was established and was funded by municipalities and the provincial government. The plan was administered by the Special Medical Relief Division of the Ontario Medical Association. By the late 1930s 600 municipalities and 2,500 doctors were participating in the scheme, which treated approximately 50,000 patients per month (Grauer 1939). Many physicians, particularly in Ontario, were involved in treating their unemployed patients and knew first hand the difficulties that their patients were facing.

Table 9.1

Caloric requirements of the 1933 Ontario Medical Association dietary standard

Age group	Calories required daily
Birth to six months	720
End of six months to end of first year	1,000
From end of first year to end of fifth year	1,500
From end of fifth year to end of tenth year	2,000
From end of tenth year to end of thirteenth year	2,500
From end of thirteenth year to end of eighteenth year	3,000
Adult female	2,500
Adult male	2,800

Source: Canadian Preparatory Committee of the British Commonwealth Scientific Conference (1936).

feeding a family of five was approximately 30 percent higher than the relief food allowance established by the provincial and various municipal welfare administrations (Struthers 1991). This scientific information from a highly credible source was used by concerned public health and welfare officials, activist community groups, and groups of unemployed workers to pressure government to increase social assistance rates (Canada 1954).

As was shown in the previous chapter, while the national food supply situation was likely adequate in the 1930s, and while prices for food were at historic lows, vulnerable subpopulations, particularly the urban unemployed, struggled to find enough money to buy food. The work of activists, medical associations, and other reformers in raising unemployment relief incomes was essential for families spending, in some cases, well over half their income on food.

At this time in Canada, unlike in the United States and Britain, almost no information was available about the dietary habits and nutritional status of the population. While, as was shown in the previous chapter, dietary surveys were conducted in the late 1930s in Canada, prior to 1939 their results were largely unavailable except to a small group of experts. Therefore, with the exception of the OMA's 1933 dietary standard, authoritative scientific information played a limited role in the public policy process leading up to the establishment of the 1938 Canadian national dietary standard.

When the results of these dietary surveys became available to the public, mainly after 1939, they were used by Toronto-area activists (see Chapter 7) and the OMA nutrition committee to pressure the Ontario government for increased relief rates. As war began in 1939, men entered the army en masse, the economy began to expand rapidly, and relief rolls across Canada dropped dramatically, with the result that the cost to governments of increasing relief rates was drastically reduced (Canada 1954). For example, between 1939 and 1941 the proportion of Ontario's population receiving social assistance decreased from 9.8 percent to 1.9 percent (Struthers 1991). Ironically, it was only towards the end of the war, in 1944, with increasing wartime prosperity and an almost full-employment economy, that the Ontario government began to use the 1938 Canadian national dietary standard as the basis for food allow-ance relief payments. Meanwhile, in the mid-1930s international ef-forts to further nutrition science found that the federal government was increasingly receptive as it began to plan a national program of unemployment insurance.

International Stakeholders and the Marriage of Nutrition and Agriculture

Efforts spearheaded by the League of Nations – based largely on research conducted by John Boyd-Orr in the early 1930s in Britain – were brought to bear on many national governments by the mid-1930s. Using Stiebeling's American dietary standard, Boyd-Orr (1936) demonstrated widespread deficiencies in the British national diet – deficiencies that increased with decreasing income.

While hunger was a problem among the unemployed and poor in Great Britain, the depth and the extent of his findings concerning un-dernutrition in the British population were, as outlined in Chapter 7, scientifically incorrect as they demonstrated widespread undernutrition and dietary inadequacy among middle- and upper-class people who were clearly well fed. Boyd-Orr's research methods contributed to an over-estimate of the extent and depth of undernutrition in the British popu-lation for two reasons. First, he utilized Stiebeling's American standard, which, given the very different dietary habits in Britain and the United States (particularly in relation to quantities of meat consumed), set too high a standard for the British population. He then raised this to a "maxi-mum" standard to attain optimal health in the population (Boyd-Orr 1936). Boyd-Orr's methods increased the likelihood of finding wide-spread dietary insufficiency in Britain because his dietary standard was too high.

Unlike in Canada, where the results of dietary surveys were unavail-able in the early and mid-1930s, in Britain the results of Boyd-Orr's research were effectively used by trade unions, unemployed workers, and anti-poverty organizations to pressure the government to increase unemployment relief rates (Mayhew 1988, 456). At a time of mass unemployment, plummeting wages, and fiscal retrenchment, British government ministers "were desperately concerned to disprove links between malnutrition, ill-health and low income," and the Ministry of Health moved quickly to block publication of Boyd-Orr's research (Mayhew 1988). In spite of these efforts, the report was published internationally and widely read by the lay public as well as by members of medical and nutrition circles, including those in Canada.

Boyd-Orr's work was aggressively championed by the League of Nations' Mixed Committee on the Problem of Nutrition, which, in 1936, reported that: "There are good reasons for believing that the trend of dietary habits, particularly in countries with a Western civilization, towards a larger consumption of protective foods would coincide with a parallel evolution of agricultural production, which would in all probability benefit the rural populations of the various countries, and might also greatly contribute to a resumption of normal economic relations between the nations" (League of Nations 1936, 14).

The objective of the League's promotion of national dietary standards was twofold: (1) to increase access to food for the poor and unemployed, particularly in rural agricultural regions, and (2) to increase demand for food, which, given worldwide food surpluses, it was believed would revive international agricultural trade, leading the world out of the economic crisis. This new Keynesian-inspired marriage between nutrition and agriculture assumed, in essence, that if national governments established scientific dietary standards, and if these showed that the unemployed and poor required better diets, then this would provide reluctant governments with the "business case" for bolstering unemployment relief payments. The idea was that increasing demand for agricultural products would generate economic and trade activity. This idea hinged entirely on a Keynesian priming of the economic pump. In the 1930s moving governments, who were mainly interested in balanced budgets, to Keynesian economic thinking was an idea before its time. Until the late 1930s the federal government of Canada (like those of most other developed nations) was determined to balance budgets by holding the line on relief spending rather than by increasing it, as was implied in the League's nutrition and agricultural advice to member nations (Grauer 1939).

The League of Nations (1936, 14) advised governments to establish national nutrition councils to collect "the opinions of technical experts concerned with the various aspects of nutrition," aiming specifically to develop national dietary standards. In 1938 Canada was the first country in the world to establish a modern dietary standard, including standards for vitamins. The reasons for this had less to do with concerns about nutrition and health and more to do with the federal government's drive to establish a national employment program. As the government increasingly came to the financial rescue of the patchwork of municipal unemployment schemes across the country, it became anxious to consolidate them and to incorporate them into a national employment program. Central to this process was the need for standards of unemployment relief that would streamline and "contract, not ... expand, existing levels of expenditure" (Struthers 1983, 212).

As early as 1933, at the urging of the League of Nations, Canada had established the Canadian Preparatory Committee of the British Commonwealth Scientific Conference (CPC), with a subcommittee on nutrition that was charged with the task of developing a national nutrition council and a dietary standard (Canadian Preparatory Committee 1936).[3] The Subcommittee on Nutrition was the key federal stakeholder responsible for introducing new international nutrition research into Canada, and its high-profile membership, along with League of Nations sponsorship, gave it both prominence and credibility. This committee shaped nascent federal nutrition policy from 1935 until the formation of the CCN in 1938.

The Origins of the Canadian Council on Nutrition

The Subcommittee on Nutrition, chaired by R.E. Wodehouse, the federal deputy minister of pensions and national health, tabled a report in the summer of 1936 that summarized the world nutrition situation, evaluated the Canadian food supply, reviewed current Canadian nutrition research, and, most important, rationalized the OMA dietary standard within the context of both Boyd-Orr's research in Britain and the League of Nations' dietary standard.

[3] The Canadian Preparatory Committee included the deputy ministers of agriculture and of pensions and national health, the director of the National Research Council, and representatives from the Dominion Bureau of Statistics and External Affairs. The Subcommittee on Nutrition consisted of the deputy minister of the Department of Pensions and National Health; the chiefs of the Statistical Branch in the Department of Labour and the Agricultural Branch of the Dominion Bureau of Statistics; various representatives from the Department of External Affairs, the Department of Agriculture, and the National Research Council; and advisors from the Ontario Medical Association and Toronto's Hospital for Sick Children (Canadian Preparatory Committee 1936). Dr. Federick Tisdall was the Toronto Hospital for Sick Childrens' representative on the committee. He was a colleague of Allan Brown's and one of the inventors of Pablum.

Dr. F. Tisdall, chairman of the OMA Subcommittee on Nutrition, lead author of the OMA dietary standard, and co-author of the CPC's report (Canadian Preparatory Committee 1936, 74), dismissed the applicability of Boyd-Orr's research to the Canadian situation, stating that it "is from such a different angle than the material presented in our OMA report ... that very little comparison can be made." He went on to outline the scientific basis of the OMA standard, stating that it "is essentially the same as Stiebeling's American standard, however, being lower than usual, due to the fact that this is a relief standard where the head of the family is not working." Further, Tisdall noted that "a study of our standard from the economic standpoint shows that it is less than the recent standard issued by the League of Nations" (ibid.).

Having positioned his standard in this way, Tisdall noted that the application of the OMA relief standard would be cheaper in Canada than would the application of the League of Nations' standard (Canadian Preparatory Committee 1936, 71). Table 9.2 indicates that, using the OMA standard, food allowance costs in Toronto would have been 30 percent higher than the then-current food allowance in the city, and that using the League's standard would increase these costs by an additional 28 percent. Therefore adopting the League's standard would have raised the food allowance for those on relief in Toronto much further than if the OMA standard was adopted (Grauer 1939).

The CPC's final summary report (Canadian Preparatory Committee 1936, 65) officially adopted the OMA relief standard, advising that "the tables and data given therein present the essential features that should

Table 9.2

Food allowances (CDN $) of the City of Toronto compared with minimum adequate diet recommended by the OMA and the minimum balanced diet recommended by the League of Nations

	Milk	Fruit and vegetables	Meat and protein-rich foods	Fats	Carbohydrates	Total
City of Toronto	1.82	0.79	0.76	0.73	2.22	6.32
OMA	1.82	1.19	1.58	1.55	2.11	8.25
League of Nations	2.99	2.56	1.76	1.86	1.41	10.58

Source: Grauer (1939).

govern the selection of diets, particularly with reference to community efforts such as are represented by public assistance administration." The report went on to explain:

> The dietary budgets set by the Committee of the OMA have been tested repeatedly in families of various age compositions and have been found practical and adequate. While the need for economy in constructing these budgets has been fully recognized, the standards adopted are considered necessary to conserve the health and vigour, to promote resistance to infection and disease, to provide for normal growth in the young, and to keep the recipients fit to undertake work when it becomes available. Attention should be directed to the fact that the prices mentioned are retail prices and that municipalities buying for relief in large quantities can reduce the cost considerably. (68)

The CPC adoption of the OMA standard amounted to de facto recognition on the part of the federal government that food allowances and, therefore, relief rates in many jurisdictions were too low. By adopting the OMA standard the federal government assumed a leadership role in establishing standards for those on relief, but it avoided the greater upward pressure on relief rates that adoption of the League of Nations' standard would have caused. The adoption of the OMA standard by the CPC – an interdisciplinary, multi-ministerial committee – was an important first step in establishing a national dietary standard, although the authority of the CPC was limited both within the federal government and with respect to its ability to influence relief administrations (over which the federal government had no constitutional authority until 1940, when a national unemployment insurance program was established).

On 19 February 1938, at a special meeting chaired by the deputy minister of pensions and national health, the CPC was disbanded, the Canadian Council on Nutrition was formed, and the decision was made to establish a Canadian national dietary standard. In Britain, where by 1935 Boyd-Orr's work had been widely publicized, leading medical and nutrition scientists had worked with reformers to increase standards and to use them to pressure government to increase relief payments. While reformers were active in Canada on these economic and nutritional issues, the lack of widely available scientific information about the Canadian diet gave nutrition scientists a key role in determining the new standard.

The First Canadian National Dietary Standard

In spite of the belief among most nutritionists that hunger was a problem (especially for poor women and children), that there was a definite income gradient (with those having less income being most likely to have poor diets), and that even low- and middle-income families were spending from 30 percent to 60 percent of their income on food, they were loathe to advocate increasing incomes for these families. Instead, they advised undertaking educational policies directed at improving the nutritional knowledge of mothers.[4]

The League of Nations encouraged each national nutrition council to develop its own dietary standard as these would vary depending on differences in population energy expenditure, dietary habits, and the nutrient content of staple foods. For nutrition experts contemplating developing a standard at this time, national data on dietary habits that could be used to modify the League's standard were essential. Because these data were almost entirely lacking in Canada, in 1938 Harriet Stiebeling, who as one of the world's preeminent experts in this area was in contact with the Canadian government, advised the CPC to wait until it had more scientific data before setting a national standard (Stiebeling 1938). The committee ignored Stiebeling's advice and decided to proceed, likely because the federal government was anxious to develop a national unemployment insurance program, for which it required a dietary standard.

The small Canadian nutrition science establishment sought a national dietary standard that both conformed with the benchmark standard developed by the League of Nations (so that it might be scientifically credible) and did not place undue pressure on relief administration. The OMA standard was a reasonable compromise as it already had semi-official status and would put upward but limited pressure on existing relief rates by allowing for a smaller increase in the food allowances of those on relief.

The key figure in drafting the new Canadian standard was Dr. E.W. McHenry, who was appointed as a Canadian Council on Nutrition scientist in February 1938. CCN meeting minutes for 1938 indicate that,

---

[4] Once again, as was the case with regard to breastfeeding advice, scientists placed responsibility for solving nutritional problems on mothers. Good mothers should not work as this would interfere with breastfeeding their infants for at least the first nine months of life. Further, they should manage their food budgets more wisely and improve their cooking habits so that they might more efficiently feed their families.

throughout that year, he drafted the standards and coordinated subsequent negotiations with peers and policy makers regarding their final form (CCN 1938b). The bulk of this correspondence was with the leading nutrition scientists in Canada, although there was also some direct correspondence with Hazel Stiebeling in the United States (CCN 1938c).

McHenry engineered a compromise to lower the League's standard to conform with Canadian dietary "needs." He was well aware of the economic implications of a new dietary standard on unemployment relief expenditures, and these considerations were central to his deliberations on the issue. For example, in an early draft of the Canadian standard (CCN 1938d), it was stated:

> In relief work the lack of a suitable standard has caused a great deal of controversy. Whether a diet is considered adequate or not depends on the standard of comparison. The statement has been frequently made that a family cannot be considered properly fed unless a diet equal to the League standard is provided. Such a diet for a family of five in Toronto would cost approximately twelve dollars a week, an amount greatly in excess of that provided by relief authorities. Obviously it is of importance to determine whether this standard should be followed or whether alterations in accord with Canadian customs should be made.

McHenry's key argument for reducing the League's standard to conform with Canadian dietary practices and habits centred on lowering energy requirements for women. He argued that many European women must work, of necessity, in the fields and must spend as much energy as men. He advocated a reduction in the League's standard for women from 2,400 to 2,000 calories to adapt to these circumstances for Canadian women.

This rationalization is ironic as McHenry, in commenting on his own dietary survey results from Toronto in 1937/38, indicated that women in low-income households tended, in the face of family food shortages, to stint on their own consumption to ensure that their husbands and children received adequate nutrition (McHenry 1939). Although correspondence between McHenry and many nutrition scientists in Canada in early 1938 indicate significant disagreement over his rationale for downgrading the League standard for women, his proposed standard was adopted in the spring of 1938 (CCN 1938a) (Table 9.3).

In 1936 the OMA's presentation to the CPC rationalized using a lower standard than the League's on the grounds that it was intended as a relief standard. The calories recommended by the League for men could

Table 9.3

Caloric requirements of the 1938 Canadian Dietary Standard

Age group/category		Calories required daily
Infants		
At one month of age		500
At six months of age		800
At one year of age		1,000
Children	*Girls*	*Boys*
From end of first to end of third year	1,250	1,400
From end of third to end of sixth year	1,650	1,900
From end of sixth to end of tenth year	2,000	2,200
From end of tenth to end of twelfth year	2,250	2,400
From end of twelfth to end of fifteenth year	2,500	3,200
From end of fifteenth to end of eighteenth year	2,500	3,600
Adults		
Women		
No manual work		2,000
Housework		2,400
Pregnant, no manual work		2,400
Pregnant, with housework		2,800
Nursing		3,000
Men		
No manual work		2,400
Light manual work		2,800
Moderate work		3,300
Hard work		4,200
Very hard work		5,000

Source: McHenry (1941b, 233).

be lowered, the OMA argued, because these heads of household were, by definition, not working and therefore had lower energy needs than working men.

McHenry could not use this rationalization in 1938 as he was proposing a standard for the entire population rather than just for the unemployed and their families. However, he was aware that the basal standard for men proposed for the new dietary standard (i.e., the standard for men who were not working) would be the key benchmark for establishing relief rates in the future. The basal standard in 1938 of 2,000 calories for women was 25 percent less than the 1933 OMA standard and, at 2,400 calories it was approximately 15 percent lower than the OMA standard for men. Thus, in 1933, while the OMA had ensured that a standard greater than most relief food allowances would be accepted by the federal government, the establishment of a much lower basal standard, particularly for women, in the 1938 national standard lent powerful scientific credibility and support to relief administrations wishing to "hold the line" on food allowances for the unemployed, undermining the ability of reformers to better feed unemployed families.

Summary

The growing inability of lower levels of government to finance their burgeoning relief rolls produced a social crisis, which put pressure on the federal government to actively intervene in employment and social assistance policy. This pressure, coupled with growing relief costs, persuaded the federal government to develop a national employment strategy (including unemployment insurance) in order to increase labour productivity and to standardize relief administration with the aim of reducing its overall costs. Dietary standards were integral to this strategy because food allowances were the single largest cost item.

In terms of nutrition policy, the OMA emerged as an important domestic stakeholder in developing dietary standards. Citizens and professional organizations were hampered by the lack of information about diet and nutrition in the Canadian population in general and among the unemployed in particular. The OMA's 1933 standard was the only scientifically authoritative one publicly available for use in the Ontario and national debates over relief food allowances.

Internationally, the League of Nations was a major influence on nutrition policy making. The League's desire to develop dietary standards that would increase the demand for food and stimulate world trade was a Keynesian economic idea that fell on deaf ears in Canada and elsewhere until near the end of the Second World War, when the cost of unemployment relief became minimal. However, the federal government did heed the League's call to establish a national nutrition council, initiating the process in 1933 with the formation of the CPC. From 1933 to 1938 this committee was the key research and policy forum. It gathered Canadian nutrition research, commissioned new research, and paved the way to a Canadian national dietary standard.

Once adopted by the CPC, the OMA standard became the unofficial benchmark for developing a national dietary standard. Data on Canadian dietary habits and Canadian food composition were virtually nonexistent in 1938, and, despite Stiebeling's recommendation to delay setting a standard until more data were available, the CCN proceeded largely in response to the needs of the proposed national employment program.

The national standard was rationalized by reducing the basal require-ments for energy intake for women by approximately 25 percent (and for men by 15 percent), in spite of the fact that the few dietary surveys that had been conducted had shown that poor women were limiting their own food intakes in order to ensure that their husbands and chil-dren were better fed. Canada's first national dietary standard, although inspired by international developments in nutrition science, was actively shaped by the federal government's requirements to develop a nation-ally coordinated cost effective system of unemployment insurance.

In the volatile political climate engendered by the unemployment crisis of the 1930s, the 1938 dietary standard indicated a toughening of the federal government's stance in its rejection of the OMA's more lib-eral standard that would have resulted in fairly substantial increases in relief rates. The role of the newly emerging nutrition scientific estab-lishment in conducting and interpreting dietary surveys and in negoti-ating and setting the national standard was key to ensuring that basal standards were low enough to place only minimal pressure on relief administrations.

Canada was the first nation to develop a modern national dietary stand-ard. Very soon after it was adopted the Second World War began, cata-pulting the nation into frenetic economic activity and full employment. The new standard, though clearly rushed into service in 1938 to serve the needs of a new national unemployment system, was first used by the CCN and the Department of Health's Nutrition Services Division as a tool for planning wartime food needs not only for Canadian civilians and the military but also for the population of Great Britain (as Canada became a major supplier of food during the war). The Canadian national dietary standard, though born in an era of concern over undernutrition, was utilized to plan food distribution in an era of plenty.

Conclusion

This book investigates three basic themes in the early history of nutrition policy in Canada: adulteration and the evolution of a system of food safety, policies on breastfeeding, and the scientific and policy developments leading to a national dietary standard. These are discussed within the context of four principal cross-cutting subthemes: the safety of cow's milk, the increasing role of the medical profession in dispensing expert nutritional advice, the role of industry in shaping nutrition education and policy, and the changing dietary and health status of the Canadian population.

While legislation establishing the food safety system in Canada was in place in 1874, it took approximately thirty-five more years of legislative and civil service infrastructure development to establish an effective national system. This legislation was based on adulteration acts passed in Britain in the 1860s and 1870s and, like these statutes, more efficiently regulated the domestic and international trade in food. The Adulteration Act, 1874, was the first consumer protection law in Canada.

While Canada was an innovator in food standards legislation, in the late nineteenth century the food safety service, handicapped by an undertrained and underequipped inspectorate as well as lack of funds with which to conduct research and development, had limited ability to capitalize on this advance. This began to change in the decade following the passage of the US Pure Food Act, 1906, when the Canadian government adopted many of the new American food standards.

As well, over the next fifteen years, civil service support for the food safety system was upgraded, culminating in the passage of the modern Food and Drug Act, 1920, responsibility for which was placed under the control of the new federal Department of Health. Shifting the act to the health department was more than symbolic as it foreshadowed a health protection as opposed to a policing approach to food safety as well as an expansion of the mandate of the food safety system.

The vitamin mania of the 1920s provided manufacturers and retailers with new opportunities for adulteration, and an expansion of laboratory infrastructure was needed to detect and handle the resulting increases in vitamin-based false health claims. As well, by the 1920s the mislabelling and misadvertising of mass produced food items had begun to take the lion's share of food inspectors' time.

While the federal system of food safety was national in scope, the public health system was an uncoordinated patchwork of provincial and municipal regimes. The federal food safety system was responsible for regulating food that was traded across provincial and national boundaries as well as for the integrity of some bulk and most processed canned and packaged foods, while the various public health systems regulated local food producers, distributors, and retailers, so that the central government only had partial control over food safety.

The disjointed constitutional and organizational structure of public health activities whose purpose was to ensure food safety made it hard to develop a coordinated strategy to improve the food supply. This, in turn, limited the federal government's efforts to address the serious issue of persistently high infant mortality in the 1920s as one of the solutions to this problem, given a major shift away from breastfeeding, was to clean up the national milk supply.

By the 1920s, while the invention of increasingly safe methods of artificial feeding may have been liberating for middle-class women (who had access to expensive certified and pasteurized milk, hygienic living conditions, and vitamins), for poor women artificial feeding was still very dangerous for their babies. The efforts of pediatricians, physicians, and reformers to provide pasteurized or certified milk in urban milk depots and child welfare clinics (which were established in many Canadian cities prior to the First World War), and the efforts of municipal public health officials to clean up local milk and water supplies, were key to reducing infant mortality.

The other solution to the problem of persistent infant mortality – a solution directly under the control of the Child Welfare Division – was to provide authoritative advice on how to slow or stop the move away from breastfeeding. While the federal government had the constitutional authority to develop national campaigns to improve child health, during the interwar years it steadily lost any real authority to directly promote nutritional health messages to mothers. This was because the scientific and moral authority of physicians, most of whom were uninterested in or actively opposed to breastfeeding, had grown steadily over the decade.

The late nineteenth century had witnessed the popularization of relatively expensive artificial infant formulas, particularly in the United States. The promotion of artificial infant feeding among paying patients was central to the evolution and popularity of pediatrics and family practice in that country and, later, in Canada. Prior to the discovery of vitamins these infant formulas were extremely dangerous because, when they were all that was fed to infants, they ensured vitamin deficiency.

As the milk supply became safer, public health officials who had formerly vilified milk began touting it as an ideal protective food for children. This about-face cut away some of the traditional public health and medical support for breastfeeding. After all, if the milk supply was safe (as it was in some locations by the 1920s), and if, as the new vitamin discoveries indicated, milk was a very good supplier of vitamins, calcium, and calories, then the traditional arguments marshalled against artificial infant feeding were blunted.

It was during this time of transition in infant feeding practices that Helen MacMurchy developed and widely disseminated her national breastfeeding guidelines. Telling mothers that they had to feed cow's milk to infants over nine months of age, and in strictly admonishing them not to feed this dangerous liquid to younger infants and to keep physicians and nurses at arm's length during the nursing process, demonstrated that federal officials were aware not only that many medical professionals were opposed to breastfeeding but also that the milk supply remained unsafe.

New attitudes towards artificial feeding among public health officials, in conjunction with its increasing promotion by family physicians and pediatricians, left federal officials such as MacMurchy with few medical allies in the fight to promote breastfeeding. At the same time it is important to note that the fading of active medical support for breastfeeding also occurred because there was a very strong demand for access to safe methods of artificial feeding. In other words, many women in Canada actively sought out physicians who would help them artificially feed their babies.

Given the massive move towards artificial infant feeding, the *CMB*'s sole focus on exclusive breastfeeding (and its denial of the existence of artificial infant feeding) rendered it increasingly irrelevant. Although the correct and courageous health promotion stance taken by the Child

Welfare Division was ineffective in promoting breastfeeding among women in the 1920s and 1930s, it may have functioned as an authoritative standard that slowed the flight to artificial feeding during the interwar years.

Throughout the 1920s Canada had one of the highest rates of infant mortality among industrialized nations. It is likely that many of these infant deaths were due to the ingestion of unclean milk and water during artificial feeding. Given the secular shift away from breastfeeding, more infant deaths might have been prevented if, during the transition period when the water and milk supply was safe in some regions and unsafe in others, the division, while strongly encouraging breastfeeding, had also strongly discouraged the ingestion of cow's milk for children over nine months of age and worked with local health authorities and industry to improve the cleanliness of the cow's milk supply.

The federal government's ability to develop policy to reduce infant mortality was hindered by its complex relationship with industry. As early as 1911 the Canadian Manufacturers Association was heavily involved with the federal government in developing food standards as this required intense interaction between federal food safety officials and the food industry. With the discovery of vitamins and the growing realization on the part of many manufacturers that they could use vitamin-based health claims to boost their sales, the relationship between the government and industry became more complicated.

The food safety service saw the addition of vitamins to food as a form of deliberate adulteration. Officials in the federal Department of Health did not develop policies to fortify the Canadian food supply with vitamins until the 1950s. Until then the culture of the department was based on the preservation of natural food purity.

Intragovernmental confusion occurred when, in the 1920s, the federal Department of Agriculture discovered the marketing potential of vitamins. The department promoted Canadian food products (particularly beef and milk), in conjunction with industry. And it often used highly targeted campaigns that featured vitamin-based health claims. Increasingly, the Department of Agriculture's marketing division allied itself with the new Department of Health, utilizing professional dieticians and nutritionists for its aggressive promotion of milk.

The Division of Child Welfare's cooperation with the Department of Agriculture's Milk Utilization Branch in marketing cow's milk to mothers was at cross-purposes with its own breastfeeding guidelines, which warned about the dangers of cow's milk. As well, because the marketing strategy of the Department of Agriculture was founded on general vitamin-based health claims, particularly for protective foods, this worked against the Food and Drug Division's efforts to keep manufacturers from adulterating of food with vitamins and proliferating false vitamin-based health claims.

The basis for the Department of Agriculture's aggressive promotion of dairy and beef was the increasing predominance of animal relative to grain and vegetable production in Canada. Expansion of herds, particularly prior to supply management policies (which were not introduced until the mid-1930s, when some marketing boards were formed), created pressure to improve sales of animal-based foods by increasing exports or by changing Canadian food purchase and dietary habits through marketing campaigns. While foods other than milk and meat were also rich in vitamins (e.g., leafy green and orange coloured vegetables as well as whole wheat cereal products), these were not promoted in the same way as were dairy products and meat.

Thus, nutrition policy was dominated by food and agricultural policy. The nutrition policy making that evolved in the 1920s in various federal government departments was uncoordinated and confused. The weakness of the new Department of Health in relation to the Department of Agriculture, and the nationally fragmented authority over public health, ensured that nutritional health policy making took a back seat to the promotion of milk and meat products throughout the inter-war years.

All these policy disjunctions were exacerbated by the Depression. In the 1930s, as infant mortality rates declined, concern shifted to maternal mortality. The crisis of continuing high maternal mortality until the invention of sulphonamides in 1937 led to two major commissions in Canada, both of which advised greater medical supervision of perinatal care. The ensuing rapid medicalization of pregnancy and perinatal care, indicated by the increase in hospital births by the eve of the Second World War (at least in urban areas), further increased the role of medical professionals in directly disseminating infant feeding advice to Canadian mothers.

Stubbornly high maternal mortality rates in Canada and other industrialized nations were due to a combination of complex Depression-era factors, including an increase in illegal abortions (due in part to the illegality of contraception) and ever more abortions being performed under less than hygienic conditions (the cause of death most often cited in the maternal mortality commissions in the 1930s). This was the result of families under economic pressure attempting to limit both fertility and physician and other birth attendants over-interference in birthing in the pre-antibiotic era.

With the growing concern over maternal mortality in the 1930s, mothers were encouraged to birth in hospitals. Yet, as the figures from the early 1930s demonstrate, at least for Ontario, maternal mortality was higher for women who birthed in hospitals than for those who did not. The increases in maternal mortality rates directly undermined breastfeeding because they led to increased morbidity, which, in turn, limited the ability of ill mothers to feed naturally. Thus, the increased medicalization of birthing in the 1930s functioned to further undermine federal efforts to promote breastfeeding.

As noted in the Department of Health reports from this time, sharpened economic competition during the 1930s increased the incidence of adulteration, mislabelling, and misadvertising. The Department of Agriculture and Canada's farmers also felt the pressure of sharpened competition as, following passage of the Smoot-Hawley Act, 1930, the US border was closed, increasing the glut of food on the Canadian market.

The health status of the population improved dramatically during the Depression. Both Apple and McKeown postulated that increased access to food mediated the relationship between changes in socio-economic conditions and health. In spite of severe economic dislocation, the peculiar agri-economic situation of the Depression led to a stable domestic food supply for most basic commodities, at least at the national level, and historically low food prices. Deflation, in combination with food abundance, likely minimized the potential impact of economic dislocation on the working poor and the unemployed as did the massive intervention by the federal government in the direct and indirect provision of relief, as well as the efforts of reformers to increase relief rates.

The evidence from the few dietary surveys conducted at the end of the Depression is limited. At the time, in comparison with the 1938 standard, wealthier families ate better than poorer ones, within poor working families men had better diets than women and children, and women and children had significant deficiencies for calcium and most vitamins. Evidence of this type is not available for the years when the Depression was most intense, from 1930 to 1934, and is not available for the unemployed. However, while many families were food insecure, based on evidence from nutrition deficiency disease mortality, it is likely that the dietary conditions faced by the poor and unemployed were actually better in the 1930s relative to the 1920s.

These dietary surveys also show that women in poor working families may have had insufficient vitamin and mineral intakes because, as mothers, they denied themselves food in order to better feed their children. Even if, with hindsight, the extent of vitamin deficiency for women in poor families was less than was thought at the time, it is clear, also from the historical record, that many poor and unemployed people in Canada waged a difficult emotional and economic struggle to feed their families (Burton 2001).

From an evaluation of trends in nutritional deficiency disease mortality in the 1930s, there is further evidence that, while some of the population may have been hungry, health-compromising malnutrition was declining nationally. The evidence, while crude, shows that deaths from non-rickets nutritional deficiency diseases remained extremely rare and constant even as the Depression deepened. All infant deaths, as well as those from rickets, declined dramatically over the decade. And, death rates from major killers of adults (tuberculosis, other infectious diseases) declined dramatically through the 1930s, while at the same time adult diseases of affluence, particularly coronary heart disease, rose dramatically.

The rapid decline in infant and rickets mortality in the 1930s cannot possibly be due to increases in breastfeeding; rather, it must have been due to the fact that conditions for artificial feeding had improved. This would have been facilitated through the wider availability of better quality and cleaner cow's milk and water as well as through better access to food for each infant. Both these factors would also account for the rapid decline in rickets mortality, as would a third factor: feeding infants cod-liver oil. It is also likely that the relative impact of these factors on reduced infant and rickets mortality would have been different in different regions of the country and even within different regions of each province.

For the urban poor and landless people living in rural areas, greater access to charity (either in the form of money or food aid) or to income determined whether a person was hungry or not. In terms of the availability of charity, early in the Depression reluctant governments became directly involved in the distribution of cash and food relief to the unemployed. In both urban and rural Canada these relief efforts were often supplemented by private charity organizations.

Given high agricultural production through the 1930s, lack of income was the main obstacle between the unemployed and access to food. For these people, their ability to acquire food depended on the relief rate, which, particularly early in the 1930s, varied widely across municipalities. Thus, among the unemployed, the relief rate was central to their ability to eat properly.

The successes of reformers in obtaining more money for the unemployed were key to reducing the very high proportions of income that poor Canadian families spent on food in the 1930s. Unemployed families were engaged in a finely balanced struggle to stave off hunger. The combination of cheap food in good supply, political pressure for direct food aid, and increases in relief payments, often won in bitterly fought battles at the municipal level, limited the size and extent of exposure to health-threatening poor quality diets among the poor and unemployed.

The role of leading nutrition scientists in improving the lives of Canada's unemployed at this time was ambiguous. First, many of the nutrition scientists who conducted the dietary surveys in Canada at the end of the 1930s were convinced that malnutrition was widespread in the population. Yet, they reverted to "blame the mother" strategies calling for mothers to use their existing funds more wisely in the purchase and preparation of food rather than calling for creating initiatives to put more income in the hands of the unemployed.

The CPC's adoption of the OMA's dietary standard was a relatively conservative response to the increasingly aggressive calls for higher dietary standards from some medical experts and citizens organizations concerned about the health of unemployed people as it was lower than both the emerging scientific benchmark standards established by the League of Nations in 1935 and Stiebeling's American standard. While adoption of the OMA standard placed political pressure on local relief administrations to raise rates, and while it showed leadership by members of the Ontario medical profession, the government's motivation was less to improve health and more to develop a standard to ensure the efficiency of the soon-to-be-established unemployment insurance system.

The unemployment crisis led to near bankruptcy for lower levels of government and drove the federal government's efforts to establish a national unemployment insurance system, which was why the government became interested in establishing a national dietary standard. The federal government's interest in a national unemployment program occurred as the League of Nations encouraged member states to develop national nutrition councils, with the specific purpose of setting dietary standards.

The OMA standard was the only authoritatively scientific standard in place in Canada in the mid-1930s, and, as such, it provided support for reformers trying to move relief rates higher. The work of physicians who developed the OMA standard placed direct upward pressure on relief administrations to increase the food allowance for the unemployed.

The 1938 adoption of a much lower basal standard effectively negated this advance in nutritional standards and ensured that arguments based on the education of mothers would be central to efforts to improve the nutritional status of the population.

There are five main lessons to be learned from this historical overview of food security and nutrition policy making in Canada. First, as noted by Riches et al. (2004) in a recent case study, Canada lacks a "joined up food and nutrition policy" in which nutrition and nutritional health policy is empowered relative to food and agricultural policy. As this book demonstrates, Canada had developed some nutrition policies by the late 1930s, but these were dominated by other central government concerns, in particular by those of the Department of Agriculture. For example, in the 1920s, although the Child Welfare Division of the Department of Health worked in alliance with the Department of Agriculture, the marketing of protective foods dominated nutritional and health policy objectives to such an extent that expensive and bacteria-ridden milk was aggressively promoted to Canadian mothers in spite of the obvious health risks. This in a nation that was rapidly moving away from breastfeeding, and at a time when unsafe milk was common in many regions of the country.

This lack of joint and coherent health messaging for milk was exacerbated by the disjunction between nutrition policy makers, who operated within the federal government, and locally based public health officials. In some regions of the country (e.g., Toronto) the milk supply was clean; in others it was disease-ridden and dangerous. While the Division of Child Welfare and the Department of Agriculture were promoting milk consumption to children over nine months of age, they seem to have been unaware of, or unconcerned with, the unevenness of municipally based governance and enforcement of milk regulations across the country.

Lack of a joint food and nutrition policy in the 1920s and 1930s meant that less than ideal nutrition education messages were developed around breastfeeding and that these were shaped more by the needs of the agricultural economy than by the issue of high infant mortality. This was exacerbated by the weakness of the federal Department of Health relative to the Department of Agriculture as well as by the lack of a strong federal public health voice. In the 1920s, nutrition policy was subordinate to food policy.

The most dominant and most coherent policy developed and widely disseminated during the interwar years concerned the aggressive promotion of milk and meat. Yet as research from the Department of

Agriculture as early as the mid-1930s showed, the main barrier to the inclusion of these foods in diets was lack of income. It was clear that poor and unemployed people, even in an economic climate where food was relatively cheap, did not purchase these foods often. The only realistic way to increase purchase of these foods would have been to put more money in the hands of poor and unemployed families yet this policy was actively opposed by the emerging nutrition science establishment in Canada on the eve of the Second World War.

The second lesson to be learned from this overview is that modern dietary standards were developed in order to feed people more, not less, food. They originated as a scientific tool specifically designed to encourage agri-economic development and world trade in a two-step process. In the first step, farmers were to move to modern, value-added farming methods by shifting from plant to animal production in order to increase the supply of protective foods. In the second step, as shown by Boyd-Orr in Britain in the mid-1930s, dietary standards, used in conjunction with dietary surveys, would demonstrate that most of the population was underfed. These observations would create the moral and scientific momentum to provide more animal-based (i.e., "protective") foods to large sections of the population in the industrial nations. The resulting revival of international agricultural trade would pull the world out of economic crisis.

The modern standard was, at its inception, designed to increase animal-based agricultural production by shifting the diets of ordinary people towards the consumption of animal fats and protein. This linkage was bolstered as agriculture expanded in the post-Second World War period and as new alliances were developed between nutrition science and agriculture. Nutrition science and its role in modern national nutrition policy making originated within the crucible of this agri-economic dynamic and the impression that malnutrition was much more widespread throughout the population than it really was. These dynamics underpinned the development of dietary standards and dietary guidelines through the Post-Second World War decades that helped the population "eat more." With rising concerns over obesity however, the current problem facing nutrition policy makers is how to offer "eat-less" advice and policy.

A new approach is likely needed – one that reconceptualizes and reconfigures the relationships among agricultural policy, nutrition policy, and health. Norway took such an approach in the late 1970s (Milio and Helsing 1998; Norum et al. 1997; Ringen 1977). In that country agricultural policy has been explicitly linked to national health and dietary goals.

The third lesson to be learned relates to the very different sets of international conditions that now face the Canadian government as it moves to develop dietary and nutritional standards. In the 1930s, the League was cognizant of the importance of national differences in diets and encouraged development of different dietary standards based on these differences. Thus, nations could develop unique standards and dietary guidance for their own populations that would lead to collective improvements in world trade and health.

In the 1930s, markets for agricultural products were closed. At present they are increasingly de-regulated and global in nature. Corporations seek trade and manufacturing efficiencies, which in turn lead to harmonization of standards and the erasure of national differences in dietary habits and preference. Governments may be in a much weaker position now than in the past if they attempt to ensure that the unique dietary needs of their populations are reflected in new trade and food safety standards.

A fourth lesson is that as newer population health frameworks demonstrate and as the fight against tobacco smoking also shows, multidimensional strategies are essential to get people to change their behaviour in health improving fashion. Health promotion efforts based solely on educational strategies tend to be taken up more quickly and easily by well educated people. The less educated and affluent members of society, usually those with the greatest health needs, are often less amenable to single strategy health promotion campaigns based solely on education.

And, as was demonstrated, in the 192 [*Is ActNow just an educational Campaign?*] tion campaigns undertaken in isolation posed by the domination of food polic marketing campaigns designed to pro nutrition education, conducted in isola side the framework of joint food and nutrition policy making, and outside of a realistic understanding of counter messaging, was overwhelmed by the market. Further, it placed too much pressure on mothers both for the difficult nutritional situation in their families and for their failure to fix it. Through the interwar years mothers were blamed by physicians for not being able to breastfeed and by MacMurchy and her officials (who also severely criticized them for working outside the home) for not breastfeeding enough. Mothers, through the interwar years, were the primary targets for all nutrition marketing campaigns by industry and agriculture. In the 1930s nutrition scientists told poor mothers that they should make do with their limited incomes and simply learn to shop and cook more efficiently even as research from the Department of Agriculture showed clearly that lack of income was the problem.

Multi-pronged strategies must be developed for modern nutrition policy making to be effective. These strategies must be based on a sociological and historical understanding that conceptualizes the holistic links between the ways in which industry, agriculture, and government operate to grow, process, distribute, sell, and regulate food products. They must also be developed along with policy, which also seeks to alter structural barriers and resolve often unstated conflicts between policy makers in agriculture and health. As well, strategies should be developed that do not run the risk of blaming individuals for failure to achieve policy goals.

The fifth lesson to be learned is that, given the steady rollback of the welfare state and the rise of food banks since the early 1980s, and given that people have much less ability to grow their own food now than they did in the 1930s, the impact of future economic crises on dietary status and nutritional health may be much more severe than it was during the Depression. In other words, with greater urbanization and increased dependence on highly concentrated markets, the ability of poor Canadians to cope with the prolonged lack of access to food attendant on any future economic crisis may be highly compromised.

References

Allen, R. 1971. *The Social Passion: Religion and Social Reform in Canada, 1914-28.* Toronto: University of Toronto Press.

American Newspaper Readership Survey. 2001. Readership Institute Media Management Center at Northwestern University, Evanston, IL. Available at http://www.readership.org.

Ames, H.B. 1972. *The City Below the Hill.* Toronto: University of Toronto Press.

Anctil, H., and M.-A. Bluteau. 1986. *Santé Société. La Santé et l'assistance publique au Québec, 1886-1986.* Québec: Bibliothèque nationale du Québec.

Apple, R.D. 1987. *Mothers and Medicine: A Social History of Infant Feeding, 1890-1950.* Madison: University of Wisconsin Press.

–. 1995. "Constructing Mothers: Scientific Motherhood in the Nineteenth and Twentieth Centuries." *Social History of Medicine* 8 (2): 161-78.

Arnup, K. 1994. *Education for Motherhood: Advice for Mothers in Twentieth-Century Canada.* Toronto: University of Toronto Press.

Baumslag, N., and D.L. Michels. 1993. *Milk, Money, and Madness: The Culture and Politics of Breastfeeding.* Westport, CT: Bergin and Garvey.

Beaton, G. 1981. "Nutritional Conditions in Canada." In *Nutrition in the 1980s: Constraints on Our Knowledge,* ed. E.D. Selvey and N. White, 221-35. New York: Alan R. Liss, Inc.

Begley, A., and G. Cardwell. 1996. "The Reliability and Readability of Nutrition Information in Australian Women's Magazines." *Australian Journal of Nutrition and Diet* 53 (4): 160-66.

Bernier, J. 1989. *La médecine au Québec: Naissance et évolution d'une profession.* Quebec: Les presses de l'université de Laval.

Bideau A, B. Desjardins, and H. Pérez-Brignoli. 1997. *Infant and Child Mortality in the Past.* Oxford and New York: Oxford University Press.

Bliss, M. 1987. *Northern Enterprise: Five Centuries of Canadian Business.* Toronto: McClelland and Stewart.

Boyd-Orr, J. 1936. *Food, Health and Income.* London: Macmillan.

Breeze, E. 1926. "Little Mothers' League." *Canadian Nurse* 22 (4): 199-200.

Britnell, G.E., and V.C. Fowke. 1962. *Canadian Agriculture in War and Peace, 1935-1950.* Stanford: Publications of the Food Research Institute, Stanford University Press.

Brown, A. 1919. "The Relation of the Pediatrician to the Community." *Public Health Journal* (later *Canadian Journal of Public Health*) 10 (2): 49-55.

–. 1931. "Preventative Paediatrics and Its Relation to the General Practitioner." *Canadian Medical Association Journal* 24: 517-22.

–. 1933. "The Prevention of Neonatal Mortality." *Canadian Medical Association Journal* 29: 264-68.

–, and G.A. Davis. 1921. "The Prevalence of Malnutrition in the Public School Children of Ontario." *The Public Health Journal* 12 (2): 66-72.

Burns A.Y. 1967. "The Child and Maternal Health Division of the Department of National Health and Welfare." *Medical Services Journal of Canada* (April): 688.

Burton P. 2001. *Marching as to War: Canada's Turbulent Years, 1899-1953*. Canada: Anchor.

Campbell, G. 1932. *Report on Provincial Policy on Administrative Methods in the Matter of Direct Relief in Ontario*. Toronto: Queen's Printer.

Canada. 1907. Meat and Canned Foods Act.

–. 1914. Dairy Industry Act.

–. 1919. Department of Health Act, S.C., c24.

–. 1920. Food and Drug Act, S.C. c27.

–. 1954. *Report of the Royal Commission on Dominion-Provincial Relations*. Ottawa: Queen's Printer.

Canadian Council on Child Welfare. 1930. "Breast Feeding Continues to Decline." *Canadian Child Welfare News* 6 (1): 29-30.

Canadian Council on Nutrition (CCN). 1938a. "A Résumé of Papers Presented at the Meeting of the National Council on Nutrition, Ottawa, 20 April." *National Health Review* 6 (22): 48-64.

–. 1938b. All Meeting Minutes obtained from Health Canada (Nutrition Division).

–. 1938c. Letter from Stiebeling to McHenry dated March 6th, 1938. Meeting Minutes obtained from Health Canada (Nutrition Division).

–. 1938d. Draft version of the 1938 Canadian Dietary Standard written by Dr. E. W. McHenry (date 1938 but no month). All Meeting Minutes obtained from Health Canada (Nutrition Division).

Canadian Preparatory Committee of the British Commonwealth Scientific Conference. 1936. "Report of the Sub-committee on Nutrition." *National Health Review* 4 (15): 57-94.

Chandler, A. 1929. "Breast Feeding in Health Centres." *Canadian Nurse* 25 (11): 663-670.

Cohen, R., and J. Heimlich. 1998. *Milk: The Deadly Poison*. New York: Argus Publishers.

Comacchio, C.R. 1993. *Nations Are Built of Babies: Saving Ontario's Mothers and Children, 1900-1940*. Montreal: McGill-Queen's University Press.

Couture, E. 1939. "The Maternal Situation in Canada." *National Health Review* 7 (24): 12-21.

–. 1940. "The Health of Mothers and Children." *National Health Review* 8 (31): 204-13.

Curran, R.E. 1954. *Canada's Food and Drug Laws*. New York and Chicago: Commerce Clearing House.

Davidson, A. 1949. *Food and Drug Administration in Canada*. Ottawa: Department of Health and Welfare.

Davison, K., and S. Guan. 1996. "The Quality of Dietary Information on the World Wide Web." *Journal of the Canadian Dietetic Association* 57 (4): 137-41.

Department of Agriculture. 1926. *Annual Report*. Ottawa: King's Printer.

–. 1927. *Annual Report*. Ottawa: King's Printer.

–. 1930. *Annual Report*. Ottawa: King's Printer.

–. 1931. *Annual Report*. Ottawa: King's Printer.

–. 1932. *Annual Report*. Ottawa: King's Printer.

–. 1933. *Annual Report*. Ottawa: King's Printer.

–. 1934. *Annual Report*. Ottawa: King's Printer.

–. 1935. *Annual Report*. Ottawa: King's Printer.

–. 1936. *Annual Report*. Ottawa: King's Printer.

–. 1937. *Annual Report*. Ottawa: King's Printer.

–. 1938. *Annual Report*. Ottawa: King's Printer.

–. 1939. *Annual Report*. Ottawa: King's Printer.

Department of Health. 1921. *Health Department Annual Reports*. Ottawa: King's Printer.

–. 1922. *Health Department Annual Report*. Ottawa: King's Printer.

–. 1923. *Health Department Annual Report*. Ottawa: King's Printer.

–. 1924. *Health Department Annual Report*. Ottawa: King's Printer.

–. 1925. *Health Department Annual Report*. Ottawa: King's Printer.

Department of Health and Social Services. 1980. *Inequalities in Health: the Black Report*. London: HMSO.

Department of Pensions and National Health. 1926. *Health Department Annual Reports*. Ottawa: King's Printer.

–. 1927. *Health Department Annual Report*. Ottawa: King's Printer.

–. 1928. *Health Department Annual Report*. Ottawa: King's Printer.

–. 1929. *Health Department Annual Report*. Ottawa: King's Printer.

–. 1930. *Health Department Annual Report*. Ottawa: King's Printer.

–. 1937. *Health Department Annual Report*. Ottawa: King's Printer.

–. 1942. *Health Department Annual Report*. Ottawa: King's Printer.

Dodd, D. 1991. "Advice to Parents: The Blue Books, Helen MacMurchy, MD, and the Federal Department of Health, 1920-34." *Canadian Bulletin of Medical History* 8: 203-30.

Dominion Bureau of Statistics. 1921-51. *Vital Statistics* (1st-30th Annual Reports: Causes of Death by Sex and Age in Canada). Ottawa: King's Printer.

–. 1926-39. *Canada Year Books*. Ottawa: King's Printer.

–. 1960. *Urban Retail Food Prices, 1914-1959*. Ottawa: Queen's Printer.

Dormandy, T. 2000. *The White Death: A History of Tuberculosis*. New York: New York University Press.

Drummond, W.M., W.J. Anderson, and T.C. Kerr. 1966. *A Review of Agricultural Policy in Canada*. Ottawa: Agricultural Economics Research Council of Canada.

Dupuis, E.M. 2002. *Nature's Perfect Food: How Milk Became America's Drink*. New York: New York University Press.

Fallows, S.J. 1988. *Food Legislative System of the UK*. London: Butterworths.

Fildes, V.A. 1986. *Breasts, Bottles, and Babies*. Edinburgh: Edinburgh University Press.

Flexner, Abraham. 1910. *Medical Education in the United States and Canada*. New York: Carnegie Trust.

Floud, R., K. Wachter, and A. Gregory. 1990. *Height, Health and History: Nutritional Status in the United Kingdom, 1750-1980*. Cambridge: Cambridge University Press.

Food and Agricultural Organization. 1996. Report of the World Food Summit, Rome. Available at http://www.fao.org/docrep/003/w3613e00.htm.

French, M., and J. Phillips. 2000. *Cheated Not Poisoned? Food Regulation in the United Kingdom, 1875-1938*. Manchester: Manchester University Press.

Friesen, G. 1987. *The Canadian Prairies: A History*. Toronto: University of Toronto Press.

Gagan, D., and R. Gagan. 2002. *For Patients of Moderate Means: A Social History of the Voluntary Public General Hospital in Canada, 1890-1950*. Montreal: McGill-Queen's University Press.

Goldberg, J.P. 1997. "Nutrition Research in the Media: The Challenge Facing Scientists." *Journal of the American College of Nutrition* 16 (6): 544-50.

–. 2000. Nutrition Communication in the 21st Century: What Are the Challenges and How Can We Meet Them?" *Nutrition* 16 (7/8): 644-46.

Goldbloom, A. 1924. "Modern Tendencies in Infant Feeding." *Canadian Medical Association Journal* 14 (8): 709-12.

–. 1945. "A Twenty-Five Year Retrospective of Infant Feeding." *Canadian Nurse* 41 (4): 279-84.

Grauer, A.E. 1939. *Public Assistance and Social Insurance: A Study Prepared for the Royal Commission on Dominion-Provincial Relations*. Ottawa: King's Printer.

Hanna W.J. 1917. *Report of the Milk Committee: Milk Committee, Food Controller for Canada*. Ottawa: King's Printer.

Hassall, A.H. 1855. *Food and Its Adulterants*. London: Longman Brown Green and Longman.

Heagerty, J. 1928. *Four Centuries of Medical History in Canada*. Vol. 1. Toronto: Macmillan, 1928.

Health and Welfare Canada. 1990. *Nutrition Recommendations: Report of the Scientific Review Committee*. Ottawa: Queen's Printer.

Hertzman, C., S. Kelly, and M. Bobak, eds. 1996. "East-West Life Expectancy Gap in Europe: Environmental and Non-Environmental Determinants." NATO ASI Series no. 2 (Environment). Vol. 19. Dordrecht: Kluwer Academic Publishers.

Heymann, J., C. Hertzman, M.L. Barer, and R.G. Evans. 2005. "New Evidence and Enhanced Understandings in Healthier Societies: From Analysis to Action." Oxford: Oxford University Press.

Hollingsworth, J.B. 1925. "Milk and Dairy Inspection." *Public Health Journal* 16 (5): 223-26.

Hoppa R.D., and T.N. Garlie. 1998. "Secular Changes in the Growth of Toronto Children during the Last Century." *Annals of Human Biology* 25 (6): 553-61.

Horn, M. 1972. *The Dirty Thirties: Canadians in the Great Depression*. Toronto: Copp Clark.

Hunter, G., and L.B. Pett. 1941. "A Dietary Survey in Edmonton." *Canadian Public Health Journal* 32 (5): 259-65.

Jukes, D.J. 1987. *Food Legislation of the UK*. Cornwall: Butterworths.

Katzmarzyk, P. 2002. "The Canadian Obesity Epidemic, 1985-1998." *Canadian Medical Association Journal* (commentary) 166 (8): 1039-40.

Kealey, G. 1980. *Toronto Workers Respond to Industrial Capitalism, 1867-1892*. Toronto: University of Toronto Press.

Kerr, J.M. 1935. *Need Our Mothers Die?* Ottawa: Canadian Welfare Council, Division on Maternal and Child Hygiene.

Keys, A. 1970. "Coronary Heart Disease in 7 Countries." *Circulation* Supplement 1: 11-1211.

Kouris-Blazos, A., T.L. Setter, and M.L. Wahlqvist. 2001. "Nutrition and Health Informatics." *Nutrition Research* 21 (1/2): 269-78.

Lalonde, M. 1974. *A New Perspective on the Health of Canadians.* Ottawa: Department of National Health and Welfare.

Leacy, F.H., ed. 1993. *Historical Statistics of Canada,* 2nd ed. Ottawa: Statistics Canada and the Social Science Federation of Canada.

League of Nations. 1936. *The Problem of Nutrition: Interim Report of the Mixed Committee on the Problem of Nutrition.* Report A.12.1936.II.B. Geneva.

Leitch, I. 1942. "The Evolution of Dietary Standards." *Nutrition Abstracts and Reviews* 11 (4): 509-21.

Levenstein, H. 1993. *Paradox of Plenty: A Social History of Eating in Modern America.* New York and Oxford: Oxford University Press.

Lewis, N., and J. Watson. 1991/92. "The Canadian Mother and Child: A Time-Honoured Tradition." *Health Promotion* Winter 91/92: 10-13.

Lusk, G. 1918. "Dietary Standards." *Journal of the American Medical Association* 70: 821.

MacDougall, C.S. 1925. "Malnutrition in Children of School Age." *Public Health Journal* 16 (1): 25-34.

MacDougall, H. 1990. *Activists and Advocates: Toronto's Health Department, 1883-1983.* Toronto and Oxford: Dundurn Press.

MacGregor, R. 1923. "Supplemental Feeding in Gastro-Intestinal Disturbances of the Breast Fed Infant." *Canadian Medical Association Journal* 13 (3): 179-80.

MacLeod, T.H., and I. MacLeod. 1987. *Tommy Douglas: The Road to Jerusalem.* Edmonton: Hurtig.

MacMurchy, H. 1910. *Infant Mortality: Special Report.* Toronto: L.K Cameron, King's Printer.

–. 1911. *Infant Mortality: Second Special Report.* Toronto: L.K Cameron, King's Printer.

–. 1912. *Infant Mortality: Third Report.* Toronto: L.K Cameron, King's Printer.

–. 1923. *Canadian Mother's Handbook.* 2nd ed. Ottawa: King's Printer.

–. 1929. *Rickets: Prevention and Cure.* Ottawa: Division of Child Welfare.

MacRae, R.J. 1999. "This Thing Called Food: Policy Failure in the Canadian Food and Agriculture System." In *For Hunger-Proof Cities: Sustainable Urban Food Systems,* ed. M. Koc, R.J. MacRae, L. Meugeot, and J. Welsh, 182-94. Ottawa: International Development Research Centre and the Ryerson Centre for Studies in Food Security.

Marmot, M.G., M. Bobak, and G. Davey-Smith. 1995. "Explanations for Social Inequalities in Health." In *Society and Health,* ed. B.C. Amick III, S. Levine, A.R. Tarlov, and D.C. Walsh, 172-210. Oxford: Oxford University Press.

Mayhew, M. 1988. "The 1930s Nutrition Controversy." *Journal of Contemporary History* 23: 445-64.

McConnachie, K. 1983. "Methodology in the Study of Women in History: A Case Study of Helen MacMurchy, M.D." *Ontario History* 75 (1): 61-70.

McHenry, E.W. 1934. *Studies on Canadian Diets: Comparison of Winter and Summer Diets of a Group of Sedentary Persons.* Ottawa: Royal Society of Canada.

–. 1939. "Nutrition in Toronto." *Canadian Public Health Journal*. 30 (1): 4-13.

–. 1941a. "Milk: The Protected, Protective Food." *Canadian Public Health Journal* 32 (4): 227-30.

–. 1941b. "Determinants of Nutritional Status." *Canadian Public Health Journal* 32 (5): 231-35.

McIlroy, L. 1938. "Diet in Pregnancy." *National Health Review* 6 (2): 94-5.

McKeown, T. 1976. *The Modern Rise of Population*. New York: Academic Press.

McKeown, T., and R.G. Brown. 1955. "Medical Evidence Related to English Population Changes in the Eighteenth Century." *Population Studies* 9: 119-41.

McLynn, F. 2005 [1759]. *The Year Britain Became Master of the World*. London: Random House.

Media Metrix. 2000. *Digital Media Audience Ratings*. Toronto: comScore Media Metrix Canada.

–. 2001. *Digital Media Audience Ratings*. Toronto: comScore Media Metrix Canada.

Miles, J., C. Petrie, M. Steel. 2000. "Slimming on the Internet." *Journal of the Royal Society of Medicine* 93 (5): 254-57.

Milio, N., and E. Helsing. 1998. *European Food and Nutrition Policies in Action*. WHO Regional Publications European Series No. 7, Copenhagen: World Health Organization.

Moscovitch, A., and G. Drover. 1987. "The Growth of the Welfare State in the Twentieth Century." In *The "Benevolent" State: The Growth of Welfare in Canada*, ed. A. Moscovitch and J. Alberts, 13-46. Toronto: Garamond Press.

Myres, A.W. 1979. "A Retrospective Look at Infant Feeding Practices in Canada: 1965-1978." *Journal of the Canadian Dietetic Association* 40 (3): 200-10.

–. 1981. "Breast-Feeding: A Canadian Perspective on a Global Priority." *Canadian Medical Association Journal* 125: 1078-42.

Nestle, M. 2002. *Food Politics: How the Food Industry Influences Nutrition and Health*. Los Angeles: University of California Press.

Newman, G. 1906. *Infant Mortality: A Social Problem*. London: Methuen.

Norum, K.R., L. Johansson, G. Botten, G.E.A. Bjorneboe, A. Oshaug. 1997. "Nutrition and Food Policy in Norway: Effects on Reduction of Coronary Heart Disease." *Nutrition Reviews* 55 (11): S32-S39

Ontario Department of Health. 1934. *Annual Report*. Toronto.

Ontario Medical Association. 1933. "Relief Diets." *Bulletin of the Ontario Medical Association* 1 (5): 33-41,

Oppenheimer J. 1983. "Childbirth in Ontario: The Transition from Home to Hospital in the Early Twentieth Century." *Ontario History* 75 (1): 36-60.

Ostry, A.S. 1994. "Public Health and the Canadian State: The Formative Years, 1880 to 1920." *Canadian Journal of Public Health* 85 (5): 293-94.

–. 1995a. "Theories of Disease Causation and Their Impact on Public Health in Nineteenth Century Canada." *Canadian Journal of Public Health* 85 (6): 368-69.

–. 1995b. "Differences in the History of Public Health in Nineteenth Century Canada and Britain." *Canadian Journal of Public Health* 86 (1): 5-6.

–. 2006. *Continuity and Change in the Canadian Healthcare System*. Ottawa: Canadian Healthcare Association.

Patterson, J.M., and E.W. McHenry. 1941. "A Dietary Investigation in Toronto Families Having Annual Incomes between $1,500 and $2,400." *Canadian Public Health Journal* 32 (5): 251-58.

Paulus, I. 1974. *The Search for Pure Food: A Sociology of Legislation in Britain*. Bristol: Barleyman Press.

Pellechia, M. 1997. "Trends in Science Coverage: A Content Analysis of Three US Newspapers." *Public Understanding of Science* 6: 49-68.

Peterkin, B.B. 1994. "USDA Food Consumption Research: Parade of Survey Greats." *American Institute of Nutrition* 9S (124): 1836-42.

Pett, L.B. 1942. "What's Wrong with Canada's Diet?" *National Health Review* 19 (36): 1-7.

–. 1944. "Malnutrition in Canada." *Journal of the Canadian Medical Association* 50: 9-14

–. 1972. "Canadian Nutrition around 1950." *Canadian Journal of Public Health* 63: 161-62.

–, and F.W. Hanley. 1947. "A Nutritional Survey among School Children in British Columbia and Saskatchewan." *Journal of the Canadian Medical Association* 56: 187-92.

–, C.A. Morrell, and F.W. Hanley. 1945. "The Development of Dietary Standards." *Canadian Journal of Public Health* 36 (June): 232-39.

Riches, G., A. Ostry, R. Macrae, and D. Buckingham. 2004. *Food Insecurity in Canada: A National Case Study* (Report for the Food and Agricultural Organization, Rome). Rome: Food and Agricultural Organization.

Ringen, K. 1977. "The Norwegian Food and Nutritional Policy." *American Journal of Public Health* 67 (6): 550-51.

Roland, C. 1981. "The Early Years of Antiseptic Surgery in Canada." In *Medicine in Canadian Society: Historical Perspectives*, ed. S.E.D. Shortt, 237-54. Montreal: McGill-Queen's University Press.

Rorke, R. 1916. "Infant Feeding." *Canadian Nurse* 12 (2): 67-70.

Rosen, G. 1958. *A History of Public Health*. Baltimore: Johns Hopkins University Press.

Rudolf, R.D. 1912. "Low Percentages in Infant Feeding." *Canadian Medical Association Journal* 2 (3): 173-80.

Saunders, S.A., and E. Back. 1940. *The Rowell-Sirois Commission: A Summary of the Report*. Toronto: Ryerson Press.

Schnell, R.L. 1987. "A Children's Bureau for Canada: The Origins of the Canadian Council on Child Welfare, 1913-1921." In *The "Benevolent" State: The Growth of Welfare in Canada*, ed. A. Moscovitch and J. Alberts, 95-110. Toronto: Garamond Press.

Shortt, S.E.D. 1981. *Medicine in Canadian Society: Historical Perspectives*. Montreal: McGill-Queen's University Press.

Sinclair, U. 1906. *The Jungle*. New York: Doubleday, Page and Company.

Smith, D. 2000. "Food Policy and Regulation: A Multiplicity of Actors and Experts." In *Food, Science, Policy and Regulation in the Twentieth Century: International and Comparative Perspectives*, ed. D.F. Smith and J. Phillips, 1-16. London: Routledge.

Smith, E. 1863. *Fifth Report of Medical Officer, Privy Council*. London: HMSO.

Spohn, H. 1920. "Infant Feeding." *Canadian Medical Monthly* 5 (9): 363-73.

Statistics Canada. 1983. "B1-14. Live Births, Crude Birth Rate, Age-Specific Fertility Rates, Gross Reproduction Rate and Percentage of Births in Hospital, Canada, 1921 to 1974." In *Historical Statistics of Canada*, 2nd ed. Cat. No.

11-516-XIE. Ottawa: Statistics Canada and Social Science Federation of Canada. Available at http://www.statcan.ca/english/freepub/11-516-XIE/free.htm.

–. 1983. "B35–50. Average Annual Number of Deaths and Death Rates for Leading Causes of Death, Canada, for Five-year Periods, 1921–1971." In *Historical Statistics of Canada*, 2nd ed. Cat. No. 11–516–XIE. Ottawa: Statistics Canada and Social Science Federation of Canada, 1983b. Available at http://www.statcan.ca/english/freepub/11-516-XIE/sectiona/toc.htm.

–. 1991. *Selected Infant Mortality and Related Statistics, Canada, 1921-1990*. Catalogue No. 82-549. Ottawa: Statistics Canada.

Stiebeling, H.K. 1933. *Food Budget for Nutrition and Production Programs*. US Department of Agriculture Miscellaneous Publication No. 183. Washington, DC: GPO.

–. 1938. Letter from Harriet Stiebeling to E.W. McHenry dated March 23rd. Letter obtained from the Canadian Council on Nutrition Files, Ottawa: Health Canada.

Stonehouse, E.H. 1922a. "The Production of Clean Milk." *Public Health Journal* 13 (10): 293-302.

–. 1922b. "A Safe and Clean Milk Supply." *Public Health Journal* 13 (10): 449-54.

Struthers, J. 1983. *No Fault of Their Own: Unemployment and the Canadian Welfare State, 1914-1941*. Toronto: University of Toronto Press.

–. 1991. "How Much Is Enough? Creating a Social Minimum in Ontario, 1930-44." *Canadian Historical Review* 52 (1): 39-83.

Stuart-Macadam, P., and K.A. Dettwyler. 1995. *Breastfeeding: Biocultural Perspectives*. New York: Aldine de Gruyter.

Sylvestre, J.E., and H. Nadeau. 1941. "Enquête sur l'alimentation habituelle des familles de petits-salaries dans la vie de Québec." *Canadian Public Health Journal* 23 (5): 241-50.

Szreter, S. 1988. "The Importance of Social Intervention in Britain's Mortality Decline c. 1850-1914: A Re-Interpretation of the Role of Public Health." *Society for the Social History of Medicine* 1: 1-38.

Thornton, P., and S. Olson. 1991. "Family Contexts of Fertility and Infant Survival in Nineteenth-Century Montreal." *Journal of Family History* 16 (4): 401-17.

–. 1997. "Infant Vulnerability in Three Cultural Settings in Montreal, 1880." In *Infant and Child Mortality in the Past*, ed. A. Bideau, B. Desjardins, and H.P. Brignoli, 216-41. Oxford: Clarendon Press.

–. 2001. "A Deadly Discrimination among Montreal Infants, 1860-1900." *Continuity and Change* 16 (1): 95-135.

Titmuss, R.M. 1938. *Poverty and Population: A Factual Study of Contemporary Social Waste*. London: Macmillan.

Urquhart, M.C., and K.A.H. Buckley. 1965. *Historical Statistics of Canada*. Toronto: Macmillan.

Ursel, J. 1992. *Private Lives, Public Policy: 100 Years of State Intervention in the Family*. Toronto: Women's Press.

Valverde, M. 1991. *The Age of Light, Soap, and Water: Moral Reform in English Canada, 1885-1925*. Toronto: McClelland and Stewart.

Wadhera, S., and J. Strachan. 1993. "Selected Mortality Statistics, Canada, 1921-1990." *Health Reports* 5 (20): 233-38.

Ward, W.P., and P.C. Ward. 1984. "Infant Birth Weight and Nutrition in Industrializing Montreal." *American Historical Review* 89 (2): 324-45.

Wells, A. 1926. "Little Mothers' Leagues in Manitoba." *Canadian Nurse* 22 (3): 140-44.

Wilkinson, R. 1989. "Class Mortality Differentials, Income Distribution and Trends in Poverty 1921-1985. *Journal of Social Policy* 18: 307-35.

Wilkinson, R.G. 1996. *Unhealthy Societies: The Affliction of Inequality*. London and New York: Routledge.

Williams, A.S. 1997. *Women and Childbirth in the Twentieth Century*. Stroud, Gloucestershire: Alan Sutton Publishing.

Wilton, P. 1995. "Cod-Liver Oil, Vitamin D and the Fight against Rickets." *Canadian Medical Association Journal* 152 (9): 1516-17.

Young, E.G. 1941. "A Dietary Survey in Halifax." *Canadian Public Health Journal* 23 (5): 236-40.

–. 1964. "Dietary Standards." In *Nutrition: A Comprehensive Treatise*. Vol. 2: *Vitamins, Nutrient Requirements and Food*, ed. G.H. Beaton and E.W. McHenry, 299-345. New York: Academy Press.

Index

CMB stands for *Canadian Mother's Book.*